INTRODUCTION TO NURSING

Concepts, Communication, and Calculation

CHESANNY BUTLER, PHD, RN, PHNA-BC, CNE

one-time online access code included

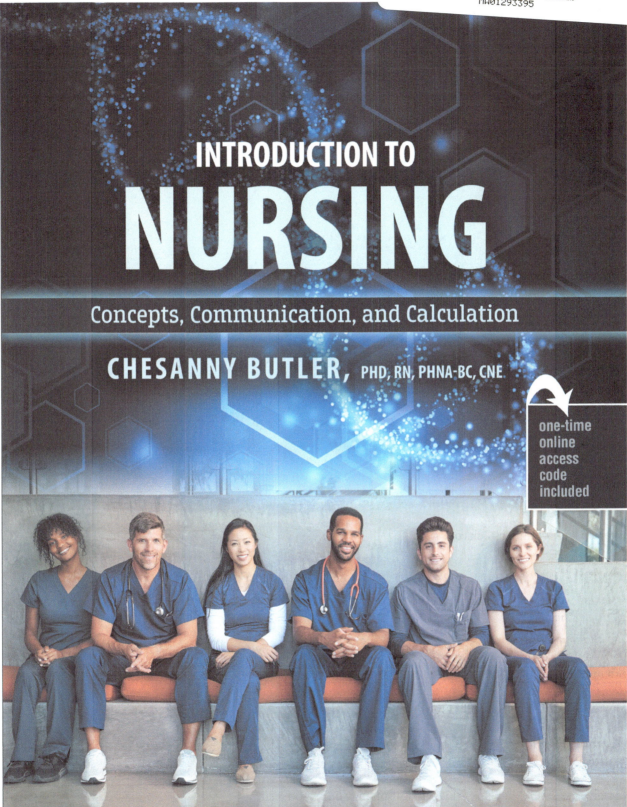

Kendall Hunt
publishing company

Cover image © Shutterstock.com

Kendall Hunt
publishing company

www.kendallhunt.com
Send all inquiries to:
4050 Westmark Drive
Dubuque, IA 52004-1840

Copyright © 2020 by Kendall Hunt Publishing Company

PAK ISBN 978-1-7924-4287-2
Text ISBN 978-1-7924-4288-9

All rights reserved. No part of this publication may be reproduced, stored in a retrieval system, or transmitted, in any form or by any means, electronic, mechanical, photocopying, recording, or otherwise, without the prior written permission of the copyright owner.

Published in the United States of America

Table of Contents

Part 1: Nursing Concepts

Chapter 1:	Introduction to the Role of the Nurse	3
Chapter 2:	An Introduction to American Nursing History	11
Chapter 3:	Professional Nursing	23
Chapter 4:	The Art and Science of Nursing	33
Chapter 5:	Foundations In Nursing Theory	53

Part 2: Nursing Communication

Chapter 6:	Patient and Health Team Communication	61
Chapter 7:	Health Literacy	83
Chapter 8:	Introduction to Medical Abbreviations	89
Chapter 9:	Introduction to Medical Terminology	97

Part 3: Nursing Calculations

Chapter 10:	Introduction to Safe Nursing Practice	131
Chapter 11:	Introduction to Medication Administration	139
Chapter 12:	Basic Math Review	161
Chapter 13:	Frequently Used Systems of Measurement	175

PART 1: NURSING CONCEPTS

Chapter 1

Introduction to the Role of the Nurse

Chapter Objectives:

- Define the nurse in health care
- Describe current nursing roles
- Discuss the important of the ANA Scope of Practice and the ANA Code of Ethics
- Compare the levels of nursing practice
- Describe the role of each level of nursing practice
- Identify the educational path and licensure of an RN
- Discuss the reasons people choose to become an RN

Have you ever wondered what kind of career you should pursue? While many people have successfully entered the field of nursing, oftentimes they wonder whether nursing is the field for them. Specifically, people wonder: What makes a good nurse? Do I like helping people? Am I caring and compassionate? Would I enjoy it? Could I make a difference in other people's lives? Let us begin with an exploration of what is meant by the term "nurse" and all of the multiple facets that make a professional nurse today.

What Is a Nurse?

Nurse, as defined by *Merriam-Webster* (2020) is "a person who cares for the sick or infirm," and yet we know that nursing is more than this. Nursing has evolved and contributes significantly to health and health care across the world. The World Health Organization (WHO, 2020) defines nursing as a field that "encompasses autonomous and collaborative care of individuals of all ages, families, groups and communities, sick or well and in all settings. It includes the promotion of health, the prevention of illness, and the care of ill, disabled and dying people." https://www.who.int/topics/nursing/en/. This definition is broader and captures the many roles of the nurse, not only for the patient but also for families and communities across the entire life span, and yet, this definition still does not reflect the "how" of nursing. In general, nursing seeks to advance the social welfare of all people through the generation and application of scientific knowledge, holistic care practice and health, disease, and wellness advocacy and education.

In the United States, The American Nurses Association (ANA) is the premiere professional nursing organization for all Registered Nurses (RNs) and is comprised of nurses interested in advancing the care and quality of care for all people. The ANA (2015) defines nursing as follows:

> "Nursing is the protection, promotion, and optimization of health and abilities, prevention of illness and injury, facilitation of healing, alleviation of suffering through the diagnosis and treatment of human response, and advocacy in the care of individuals, families, groups, communities, and populations" (p. 7).

In this definition, we begin to see a reflection of "how" nurses will respond and care. The responsibility of any professional organization is to develop the scope and standards by which the profession will practice. The ANA has accepted this responsibility and continuously works to provide these standards to ensure alignment between professionals and public safety.

As a strong professional nursing organization, the ANA provides a very clear, concise definition of what nursing is and the different types of nursing practice seen today. Nursing is complex and encompasses a wide range of holistic care practices blending both the art and science of healthcare with a strong philosophy rooted in compassion, dignity, and respect for all people. Nursing is not only a profession, but also a description of our calling; an acknowledgment of who we are in our soul. A calling can best be exemplified by discussing the emotional and spiritual component of how and why we care for people and listening to nurses describe this connection as a feeling or innate belief that they have always known in their heart that they should become a nurse. The art of nursing involves a genuine feeling in the heart, a true desire to provide comfort and peace of mind for others. Nursing is also a science. It requires critical thought, judgment, and advanced skills. Nursing, as a profession, works tirelessly to ensure nurses have the most rigorous and current education, an education and training that allows nurses to provide the most up-to-date evidence-based interventions in attempting to support patients in returning to the highest level of health possible. https://www.nursingworld.org/practice-policy/workforce/what-is-nursing/. Nursing is based on very specific core values. These values are reflected by all RNs and include the underlying principles central to nursing practice: quality care and outcomes, evidence-based health promotion and delivery, individualization, teamwork and collaboration, advocacy, use of the nursing process. We will explore each of these concepts in greater detail later in this text.

Nursing Roles

Nurses and nursing can be traced throughout history. Although those who have been identified as nurses have always had the role of caring for the infirm, the way this has been accomplished has varied greatly. Nurses have always used observation, ingenuity, tradition, and knowledge to provide as much comfort, care, and support to their patients as possible. Although we see that some people have been required to assume the role of caring for others throughout history, many have done so willingly and have sought training. We will explore a very brief but insightful history of nursing in Chapter 2 and break down the foundations of nursing so that we can better understand the role of nursing today.

In an attempt to gain public trust, ensure quality, and provide competent care practices, nursing has evolved greatly over the past 100 years to identify specific professional roles, procedures, services, and responsibilities that RNs are allowed to perform, based on competency and training, under the law. In nursing, this is referred to as the Nursing Professional Scope of Practice https://www.nursingworld.org/practice-policy/scope-of-practice/, which provides the framework, context, and required competencies in support of the standard of care. Within the nursing profession, we find two documents that form the backbone of nursing practice in the United States. The first is *The Code of Ethics for Nurses with Interpretive Statements*, which is comprised of nine ethical provisions of nursing practice that illustrate the ethical framework within which all RNs must practice. We will be focusing on what ethics are and how they are applied in nursing within Chapter 3. https://www.nursingworld.org/practice-policy/nursing-excellence/ethics/code-of-ethics-for-nurses/coe-view-only/. The second document is *Nursing: Scope and Standards of Practice, Third Edition*, https://www.iupuc.edu/health-sciences/files/Nursing-ScopeStandards-3E.pdf, which outlines the expectations of professional nursing practice.

The RN Scope of Practice provides the general public and RNs at large with a full understanding of all components of each role that professional RNs must align their practice with when caring for all patients. The ANA's *Scope of Practice* is truly the "who, what, where, when, why, and how" of nursing and provides a clear guideline.

As you can see, nursing has evolved into a very highly technical profession governed by rules and regulations to help protect the public but has never deviated from the original ideal of the provision of care. Today, given the vast range of health care services and skills, nursing roles are divided into three categories and are based on the level of legal responsibility provided to them. The Licensed Practical Nurse (LPN), the Registered Nurse (RN), and the Advanced Practice Nurse (APRN).

Registered Nurse Licensure

The Registered Nurse (RN) credentials are not bestowed on a graduate of an accredited nursing program simply by graduating. The nursing graduate, whether having graduated from a two-year program and acquired an Associate Degree in Nursing (ADN) or having completed a Bachelor of Science in Nursing from a four-year program (BSN), must still apply, complete, and pass a licensure exam to be considered a RN. The licensure exam for an RN is called the National Council Licensure Examination or NCLEX-RN. Eligibility requirements and the process for applying for the licensure exam can be found through The National Council of State Boards of Nursing website (NCSBN; https://www.ncsbn.org/NCLEX_Bulletin_March_2020.pdf).

Once a graduate nurse has passed the NCLEX-RN and successfully acquired licensure in an individual state or through the Nurse Licensure Compact, the RN must adhere to the Scope of Practice for the board/s of nursing in the state/s in which he or she is now licensed. Every state in the United States has a distinct board of nursing whose sole purpose is to ensure the protection of the public from harm. In so doing, the board is the entity that sets the requirements for initial licensure and the guidelines for licensure renewal. They also regulate the basic education requirements, competency level, and required continuing education for licensure renewal. The state board of nursing in each state is also responsible for defining the nurse practice act or scope of nursing practice within the state for general nurses and advanced practitioners and investigating any complaints made by a person or entity or agency against a licensee. The board of nursing also determines any disciplinary action that may be necessary, which can include licensure revocation or suspension. The NCSBN offers a comprehensive set of links to all U.S. State Boards of Nursing and their accompanying Nurse Practice Acts: https://www.ncsbn.org/npa.htm

> Nurse Licensure Compact: https://www.ncsbn.org/nurse-licensure-compact.htm
> NLC map of states in 2020 currently participating in multistate licensure: https://www.ncsbn.org/NLC_Map_Updated_June_2019.pdf

This means that you can practice as an RN only in specific state/s and must uphold all legal and ethical requirements contained in the standards. Because there are so many specialties and such a diverse market of RNs' employers, it is important to make sure you are fully knowledgeable regarding these regulations. Although the RN is legally covered by scope of practice in the state for which he or she is licensed, it is important to also compare job description and employer policies and procedures when working as an RN to ensure alignment and personal competency. Understand that your scope of practice contained within a policy or procedure should ever require you to practice outside of your state's Scope of Practice or that of the General Scope and Standards of Practice from the ANA.

After graduating and successfully acquiring the RN licensure, nurses generally determine what area of nursing practice they would like to work within. Currently, the United States has dozens of nursing specialties and, as discussed previously, associated professional organizations that accompany each of them. For a comprehensive list of current nursing specialties in the United States, visit https://www.purdueglobal.edu/blog/nursing/list-nursing-specialties/

A nursing specialty refers to an area of study and clinical practice that requires additional training, competency, and experience. Although some specialties require additional higher education and credentialing and fall into the category of Advanced Practice, as in the case of Nurse Midwifery, or a Family Nurse Practitioner, other specialties involve basic RN licensure such as an Emergency Room Nurse or a Home Health Care Nurse. Once an RN begins to specialize in an area of nursing, the ANA in conjunction with the State Board of Nursing also requires that you adhere to the specialty organization's Scope of Practice, which provides very specific guidelines within the specialty regarding standards of practice. Often, a certification in a specialty area is not only a way to further the RNs education, but also provides additional reassurance to the public that the nurse has the required competencies to fully provide specialty skills.

For example, a new graduate nurse does not possess the general skill set to administer intravenous chemotherapeutic agents to adult cancer patients. But if the RN is hired by an Oncology Infusion Center, the nurse is frequently required, by the employer, to obtain certifications in oncology and infusion. These certifications come with their own scope of practice and set of credentials that inform the public of the nurse's competency, experience, and knowledge to administer oncology infusion medications effectively and safely. There are two credentials that the nurse in this example would be required to obtain: (1) the CRNI® or Certified Registered Nurse Infusion and (2) the ONC® or Oncology Certified Nurse. The first certification means that the nurse is competent in the latest advances and core areas in infusion nursing, and the second certification means that the nurse has the basic competency and training to care for adult cancer patients. If you have not already guessed, RNs are lifelong learners. Within their role, they not only expect but also demand continuous education to ensure that they stay abreast of the latest procedures, regulations, skills, and evidence in practice for the well-being of the patients in their charge.

Levels of Nursing Practice and Educational Requirements

Practical Nurse (PN)

The Practical Nurse (PN), Licensed Practical Nurse (LPN), and the Licensed Vocational Nurse (LVN) are all of the same group of licensed nurses used to provide basic and routine care and support to the patient and report minor changes to their supervising RNs or other advanced health care provider. The educational requirements of an LPN can range from a certificate (after completing approximately a year of specific training) to an Associate Degree in Applied Science as is the case with some technical colleges. Although there is also a national licensure exam for the LPN, the scope of the LPN is quite different. The licensure exam for the LPN is also administered by the NCSBN and is referred to as the NCLEX. The difference is the version of the exam. The LPN licensure exam is specifically called the NCLEX-PN, which denotes "practical nurse." Comparing the level of PN difficulty (LPN or LVN) between the NCLEX-RN and the NCLEX-PN is not appropriate because each exam is designed to measure the specific knowledge, skills, and decision-making capability required for the identified role. Because the RN role carries with it direct oversight for the management and care of the patient, the NCLEX-RN exam naturally involves high levels of critical thinking, and in-depth use of the nursing process.

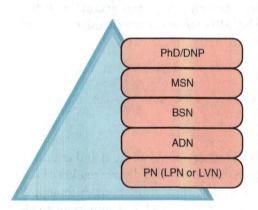

The day-to-day tasks of an LPN vary from state to state, and their scope is regulated, just like the RN's, by the state board of nursing for which they hold their license. In general terms, the LPN provides basic, necessary, and practical skilled care as well as education to patients and their families. The LPN can practice in a variety of settings and specialties and is routinely licensed to provide medications to patients, provide cardiopulmonary resuscitation (CPR), if needed, complete vital signs, change dressings, collect specimens that will be submitted to the lab, insert and maintain indwelling care supplies such as a urinary catheter, ostomy, or nasogastric tube, provide feedings and nourishments, keep a record of the patient's progress and general health as well as monitor and report clinical patient condition changes to the RN and/or provider. Depending on the state, LPNs can be found working in a number of health care settings to include hospitals, rehabilitation centers, nursing homes and long-term care agencies, home health agencies, and many medical offices and urgent care settings. To learn more about the beginning of the LPN role, visit https://www.nursinglicensure.org/articles/lvn-lpn.html

Registered Nurse (RN)

When we think of the term "nurse," the RN is generally what comes to mind. RNs are responsible for a wide range of duties and rely on all aspects of their strong education. The roles often include being an expert educator and communicator for patients and their families and also an astute researcher: participating in and improving the clinical environment and quality of patient care and developing new, more effective nursing techniques.

They must also be excellent clinicians: being able to fully assess, monitor, and create plans of care for those in their charge. They are fully responsible for the day-to-day care of the patient and must stay abreast of all new developments, including medical equipment, procedures, medication administration, blood products, diagnostic test preparation and laboratory report interpretation, team collaboration and consultation, and, above all, must have exceptional critical thinking and clinical judgment skills.

Although all RNs have some form of managerial responsibility, they must also know how to lead and manage effective patient care teams and communicate effectively with patients, families, groups, and other health care team members. RNs work together with multiple health care workers and often have oversight of LPNs, Nursing Assistants (NA), and other ancillary support staff in direct patient care. Naturally, their capabilities are driven by their education and training/certification, but where they are needed is rarely limited, especially when it comes to industries in which an RN may be employed. RNs work not only in hospitals, clinics, and agencies involved in direct patient care, but also outside of direct patient care arenas and are frequently found in legal offices, public health departments, and community liaison agencies, running independent nursing care facilities, lobbying in the political arena, working as researchers, administrators, and even as sales representatives for medical supply or pharmaceutical companies.

The educational requirements for a Registered Nurse vary by state but culminate in the NCLEX-RN licensure examination. To become an RN, a minimum of an ADN, which is a two-year degree, or a BSN, which is a four-year degree, is required. Although many people may choose to begin their RN journey using the ADN route, through a community or technical college, most employers today require the graduate to obtain a BSN within only a few short years, as a condition of employment. There has been a significant push in the United States, given the tremendous value added to patient care and safety, for 80% of all RNs to have a BSN by 2020 (IOM Report, 2011). However, for numerous reasons the progress toward this goal has remained slow, with only approximately 65% of U.S. RNs in 2020 having met this targeted goal. The new projection for reaching this goal, according to J. Spetz (2018), at the Philip R. Lee Institute for Health Policy Studies, would be 2025 (https://nepincollaborative.org/wp-content/uploads/2018/07/Spetz-2018-BSN-80-percent-forecast.pdf).

The difference between the degrees is vast. The additional education adds to the foundational knowledge of the nurse, which includes key concepts essential to full practice. These classes include the addition of training in public and community health, leadership, health care delivery systems, communication, critical thinking, additional health assessment training, and even mental health. The exact courses and requirements both in the classroom and in the clinical practice arena vary and should be carefully reviewed when looking to complete what is called the RN to BSN slide. This is the common term used to describe an educational program that allows ADN graduates who have passed the NCLEX-RN licensure exam to complete their training and obtain a Bachelor of Science Degree in Nursing.

As discussed, although many newly graduated students obtain their RN license and go on to work in a hospital setting, some may choose other practice environments. Within the direct patient care arena, however, the day-to-day responsibilities of an RN can vary and may be based on the number of years of direct patient care experience and specialization. Generally, these direct patient care responsibilities include taking care of a team of patients assigned to the RN based on the patient acuity level; performing numerous forms of physical assessments; and obtaining detailed health histories, genograms, and other specific assessments such as mental health or infection exposure risks. The RN is responsible for the development and maintenance of an individualized patient plan of care, provides counseling and education, administers medications or other nursing interventions, coordinates holistic care in collaboration with other members of the health care team, and works in tandem with the health care provider to ensure patient care, comfort, and return to an optimal state of wellness. RNs also work with case managers and coordinators to ensure a smooth transition of each patient from the direct care setting to either other facilities such as home care or back to the direct care of their primary care provider in the community. This is called continuity of care and is an essential function of the Registered Nurse.

Advanced Practice Registered Nurse (APRN)

An Advanced Practice Registered Nurse (APRN) is a category of RNs indicating that an RN has gone back to school to obtain a master's (an additional 2 years of higher education in an accredited nursing program) and/or a doctoral degree (an additional 2–4 years past the master's degree) in nursing practice. Obtaining these degrees, when pursuing a clinical track, means that the RN has the specific intention of practicing in any of the following common areas:

- Nurse Practitioner (NP): https://nurse.org/resources/nurse-practitioner/
- Clinical Nurse Specialist (CNS): https://nurse.org/resources/clinical-nurse-specialist/
- Certified Registered Nurse Anesthetist (CRNA): https://nurse.org/resources/nurse-anesthetist/
- Certified Nurse Midwife (CNM): https://nurse.org/resources/certified-nurse-midwife/
- Advanced Practice Public Health Nurse (APHN-BC): https://nurse.org/resources/public-health-nurse/.

Additionally, when the RN desires to pursue a career path in a more nonclinical role, we often see RNs pursuing roles such as the:

- Certified Nurse Educator (CNE): https://nurse.org/education/msn-nurse-educator-guide/
- Nursing Administrator (NA): https://nurse.org/resources/nurse-manager/
- Informatics Nurse Specialist (INS): https://nurse.org/articles/nursing-informatics-salary-and-career-opportunitie/

As with all lifelong learning, the goal in nursing is to always maintain the highest level of competence and continuous education. Lifelong learning ensures that nurses stay current in all aspects of patient care and can lead, educate, and develop technology to meet the demand for health care for generations to come. Many of the advanced roles in nursing require successful completion of the highest available degree. Just as a university professor, who teaches the next generation of nurses, is expected to be a true expert in his or her field, Nurse Practitioners, who medically diagnose and treat the public, are expected to have the highest level of training and treatment knowledge available to ensure correct, accurate, and safe patient management. Many of these advance roles require the individual to successfully complete a doctorate in Nursing Practice, obtained by those whose focus remains in the clinical arena in the management of patient health care. The PhD represents the prestigious Doctor of Philosophy, the highest university degree conferred by any course of study and is recognized around the world. A PhD is obtained by those who wish to advance the profession of nursing through research and scholarship.

APRN roles require continuous updating of education training, recertification, and additional licensure requirements. The guidelines for the scope of practice for each APRN are also regulated by each individual state board of nursing and must be monitored closely. Additionally, the scope of practice for each of the specialty organizations under which the APRN practices provides additional practice guidelines. An example of a specialty organization with oversight over Nurse Practitioners is the American Association of Nurse Practitioners (AANP) https://www.aanp.org.

This organization is responsible for advancing education, setting policy and advocacy agendas, and providing the latest evidence-based practice for all Nurse Practitioners nationwide.

Certain APRN roles, such as the Nurse Practitioner or Certified Nurse Midwife, may apply for prescriptive authority, which is used by the NP and CNM to write medication prescriptions for patients. This privilege comes with an extreme responsibility to ensure the safety of the public and is governed by the United States Department of Justice Drug Enforcement Administration. Any APRN who is granted prescriptive authority must apply for a DEA number, a special license that allows providers to legally prescribe medication. https://www.deadiversion.usdoj.gov/online_forms_apps.html. Special additional continuous education training is required for all APRNs with prescriptive authority.

Characteristics of Nurses

Why Do People Choose Nursing?

Although images of nurses are deeply woven into our culture through media—television, streaming movies, documentaries, and even socially through personal posts and news feeds—our idea of what a nurse is can also come from personal experiences, family, or a personal belief that we have been spiritually called to the field. For many nurses, the question why they became a nurse can be tied to one specific answer, whereas others have two or more reasons. Why do you want to be a nurse? Here are the top six reasons pervading nursing research on this topic for decades.

A Personal Experience: Have you ever heard someone say that they wanted to become a nurse because of a specific memory or moment in their life? Oftentimes, people tell stories of a nurse whose interactions with them left such a significant impression that they themselves wanted to become a nurse from that moment on. The Internet, news, and even social media are replete with stories of how a nurse changed someone's life and inspired him or her to take up the call. This usually happens either as a result of a personal patient experience or because they witnessed the care and compassion of a nurse while they were caring for a family member. While the interaction or experience can be either a positive or negative memory, the outcome is generally the same: the strong desire to go to nursing school.

A Desire to Help Other: Generally, nursing students have a reason for becoming a nurse; after all, the path is not an easy one, and the rigorous curriculum is often underestimated. A commonly cited reason seems like no real reason at all, and yet it is one of the strongest and most foundational characteristics a nurse can have: the genuine desire to help another. Stories of childhood spent bandaging their family members and playing nurse when people were sick come to mind; sharing candies as pretend pills; taking care of sick pets; or simply role-playing the nurse with young friends are all images we discuss when our reasons for wanting to be a nurse are reflected upon. As we grow up, we may realize that we need more to our story than a simple basic desire, and yet oftentimes when we say we want a stable career or a good paying job, it does not seem to have the level of significance that true desire brings forth. Having a desire to help others is part of who we are as nurses and, if asked, is one of the reasons all nurses provide when they are asked why they do what they do.

A Spiritual Calling or Knowing: In 1997, Dr. Ritva Raatikainen published a study entitled, *Nursing care as a calling*. In the study, she defines the calling to nursing that many describe as "a deep internal desire to choose a task or profession which a person experiences as valuable and considers [their] own" (Raatikainen, 1997, p. 1111).

Since the beginning of the history of nursing, we have evidence that "the call to tend the sick and infirm" has existed for thousands of nurses as the primary reason for their career path. Steeped heavily in religion and spiritual experience, we see that throughout history many nurses, both male and female, have been religious persons or have had a spiritual encounter during which the person decides to dedicate their lives to the health and well-being of the sick or injured.

The call many nurses answer can also be the call, or the response, to people in society. An example of this can be seen before, during, and after times of national crisis or war. This refers to the "call of humanity" to come forth and help people in a time of need. We know that this selfless act is one of our greatest possible gifts to each other. We have seen this "call" in media campaigns surrounding hurricanes and wildfires through agencies such as the American Red Cross and highlighted in news specials after pandemics like Covid-19. Answering the call, whether a religious calling or a response to a societal need, is a noble rationale steeped in history and is a strong part of many nursing campaigns like those from Johnson and Johnson.

A Family Member: Having a family member such as a mother, brother, father, aunt, or grandparent who is a Registered Nurse is quite common in the nursing field. Often, nursing is a generation career tradition, and we see not only a family line of professional nurses but also other members of the family who enjoy a career in some health care field. During the 21st century, we have seen up to four generations of nurses within one familial line, sometimes all working at the same hospital. For example, students who share that it is a family member that inspired them to become a nurse often also report high levels of career satisfaction and family pride in this tradition, and yet we also see that the nurses often pursue different specialties of nursing. For example, Esther Schaal, who passed away at the age of 95 in 2010, was the mother of Jane Schaal, who also entered nursing having known since childhood that nursing was what she was meant to do. Jane Schaal was followed by her daughter, Mary Jane Sage, as an RN. Not surprisingly, in December of 2019, Mary Jane Sage's own daughter, Emily Sage, graduated from nursing school and began her role as an RN. This line of nurses also happens to have all worked at the same hospital and has definitely made nursing a family career. Each person in the family was inspired both by a family influence and a personal "knowing" that nursing was his or her calling right since childhood. Video link: https://spectrumlocalnews.com/nys/rochester/coronavirus/2020/05/07/four-generations-of-nurses-answer-the-call-at-the-same-batavia-hospital?cid=share_clip

Pay/Stability: Often, we hear people say, "You should be a nurse. It is a stable career, and you will always be able to find a position." This is strong advice. Despite a traditional 5-year cyclical pattern of nurses coming and going from the market, the field of nursing affords you numerous opportunities to move within a field and across other industries. How much money does a Registered Nurse make each year? This is another very important consideration, and an additional reason people choose to pursue nursing. Although nurses make more or less, depending on education level, years of experience, and specific specialty training and certifications, nurses make a comfortable living overall. Nurse Journal is an organization that has been monitoring the pay scales in the nursing market. There are many other comparative websites, but taking a moment to explore these trends are a very important consideration for your future. https://nursejournal.org/registered-nursing/rn-careers-salary-outlook/.

Reputation: In a 2016 Gallup Poll, nursing has held the highest public rating (84%) among all professions, ranking "high" or "very high" in honesty and ethical practice. This ranking is a position that nursing has held in the hearts of Americans for the last 20 years and should not be taken lightly. https://news.gallup.com/poll/200057/americans-rate-healthcare-providers-high-honesty-ethics.aspx.

Nursing, as an art and science, has had a long-standing history of excellence in the provision of care and compassion, honesty, trustworthiness, and professional integrity. When we think of a nurse at the bedside, we think of someone who is there to listen, to provide a healing touch, and to help us through some of our most difficult days. The RN takes the time to know the patient, make connections with their families, make us smile and laugh, provide that individualized comfort, and is trusted with some of our most difficult health challenges. They are knowledgeable, advocate for people, and are fully invested in helping each person derive their best quality of life, all the while making each person feel as though he or she is the only patient in their care. The reputation of each RN is fully dependent on those who have come before them and those who accept the charge to come after them in our world. Each RN abides by the same Code of Ethics and holds each other accountable to these same standards to ensure nursing remains the most trusted, most ethical, and most compassionate discipline for generations to come.

Summary

Identifying if nursing is the correct path, for any student pursuing a field in health care, is the first step in a professional career. Defining and discovering the roles of a professional nurse as well as understanding the characteristics, values, and beliefs that nurses possess help to clarify whether nursing is the field of study for you. Professions are guided by core values and define their scope of practice as well as the ethical code they will follow to ensure competency and excellence in the provision of care. Although there have been numerous published studies over the years in which researchers have attempted to better understand the reasons people choose to become a nurse, ultimately, we, as a profession, have recognized many of the top six reasons for having remained stable despite the country of origin with regard to nursing.

References

American Nurses Association. (2015). *Nursing: Scope and standards of practice* (3rd ed.). Silver Spring, MD: Author.

Institute of Medicine. (2011). *The future of nursing: Leading change, advancing health*. Washington, DC: The National Academies Press.

Merriam-Webster Dictionary. (2020). Nurse [definition]. Retrieved from https://www.merriam-webster.com/dictionary/nurse

Raatikainen, R. (1997). Nursing care as a calling. *Journal of Advanced Nursing, 25*(6), 1111–1115. Retrieved from https://onlinelibrary.wiley.com/doi/epdf/10.1046/j.1365-2648.1997.19970251111.x

Spetz, J. (2018). Projections of progress toward the 80% bachelor of science in nursing recommendation and strategies to accelerate change. *Nursing Outlook*. Retrieved from https://doi.org/10.1016/j.outlook.2018.04.012

Chapter 2

An Introduction to American Nursing History

Chapter Objectives:

- Define the four philosophical periods that align with nursing history
- Describe the events in each historical period that shaped the development of nursing
- Describe how nursing responds to societal change and need
- Describe the contributions made by selected nurses in American history
- Identify the increasing preparation and training required for nurses
- Identify important contributions to nursing by decade
- Discuss future nursing roles

Nursing encompasses a broad history that spans many generations of caring for the sick, injured, poor, and destitute. Early nurses were anyone, both men and women, who had a desire to help others often, without formal training. As the practice of nursing developed, many women trained to become nurses as a lifetime career, choosing to remain single to devote themselves entirely to their profession. The advances that nurses through history have made within their field have helped to bring people of all different backgrounds into this important career. Nurses have responded and always will respond to the needs of their patients. This is the key to why we study history. We know that nursing was created out of and continues to be shaped by social, political, religious, and global issues. We need to listen to this story so that we can anticipate the needs of people tomorrow. In times of war, nurses responded by meeting the needs of the wounded in combat zones and military hospitals in the United States and abroad. When communities face health care crises, such as disease outbreaks or insufficient health care resources, nurses establish community-based immunization and screening programs, treatment clinics, and health promotion activities. Patients are most vulnerable when they are injured, sick, or dying. Today, nurses are active in determining best practices in a variety of areas such as skin care management, pain control, nutritional management, and care of individuals across the life span. Nurse researchers are leaders in expanding knowledge and developing innovation in nursing and other health care disciplines. Their work provides evidence for practice to ensure that nurses have the best available evidence to support their practices. Knowledge of the history of the nursing profession increases your ability to understand the social and intellectual origins of the discipline. Although it is not practical to describe all of the historical aspects of professional nursing, some of the more significant nursing leaders and milestones are described here to give you an introduction to where nursing has been, where we are now, and where we are destined to go in the future.

Bevis (1989) categorizes history into four philosophic periods, which coincidentally align with the reasons people choose nursing, discussed in Chapter 1: asceticism, romanticism, pragmatism, and humanistic existentialism (p. 36).

Asceticism

Asceticism occurred during the time of classicism and Plato, in the third century AD, when people were focused on denying physical and psychological desires in an attempt to achieve higher-level spiritual guidance and ideals; resisting temptation and immediate impulsivity. This was a time of discipline and endurance in mental, physical, moral, and spiritual achievement and was a hallmark of the creation of many religions (*Encyclopedia Britannica*, 2020). https://www.britannica.com/topic/asceticism.

As early as 475 to 1500 BC, nurses during these Middle Ages were mostly women who were untrained and helped with the delivery of babies or provided service as wet nurses. Learning how to become a nurse came in the form of on-the-job training, where hard work did not come with monetary remuneration. Formal "nurses" were often nuns who were called to care for the sick and the poor as a religious calling and received no compensation; rather, it was considered the correct path as a spiritual, higher order ideal of charity. In 1113, The Knights of Malta began an "Order of the Hospital" on the island of Malta, as a work of hospice. The order was sanctioned by Pope Paschal II and dedicated to St. John the Baptist. During this time, the establishment of a hospital concept was developed, but solely for the care of those who were dying or destitute. One hundred years later, in 1247, a new direction in health care emerged, as Bethlem Royal Hospital opened in London as an institution to care for those with mental illness. This direction in care was not born out of compassion but rather as a means to remove "disturbed and dangerous" individuals from society and experiment with proposed treatments. The hospital has remained open for over 750 years and was nicknamed "bedlam." Bedlam in the English language today has come to mean "a state of uproar and confusion" (*Merriam-Webster*, 2020).

This notion of nursing as a calling and not as a paid role prevailed well into the 20th century. Today, nurses are still expected to "work for free" in donating their skill and time charitably to community and cause.

Romanticism, the second philosophical period (1798–1870), was born out of the industrial revolution and a time of materialistic idealism. Despite the meaning of the word, the period was not defined by love, but represented a complete shift in the way people thought of themselves and society. In this period, the emphasis was on an escape from realism, as a reaction to the classical period, where inspiration, subjectivity, and fantasy formed ideals. In a time of great innovation in industry and artistry in both music and visual expression, nurses depended on the physician and lacked autonomous and independent roles. The period was dotted with poetry, symbolism, and myth, as well as the journaling of nurses who aspired, intentionally or out of societal need, to function more as physicians. Such roles included midwives and apothecaries. Nurses recorded many observations, such as Florence Nightingale's *Notes on Nursing*. Additionally, several adventures of nursing stories were written during this time, romanticizing the role of nurses until well into the 20th century. This included the nursing image of the handmaiden and the civil war's urgent pleas for women's help in caring for the wounded. Although nursing formalized training at the time paralleled medical content on disease, the "lady-of-the-house" role was assumed in hospitals at the time by nurses and students, who reported directly to hospital administrators and physicians.

Pragmatic Period (World War I to end of World War II)

Pragmatism represented a period of history when truth and precise meaning were paramount. Daily life and its subsequent success depended on the practical application of all matters. This philosophical change was brought about by World War I (WWI), in 1914, and lasted till the end of World War II (WWII), in 1945. During this time, resources were scarce, including people and money, and this was exacerbated by the U.S. stock market crash of 1929. Low wages, significant debt, large bank loans, and an inadequate agricultural sector led to an ideal of penny pinching and necessity only. Nursing responded to this hardy climate with the creation of women in military nursing roles; the creation of practical nurses, aides, and technicians; the continuation of religious nursing vocation; and the creation of several women's auxiliaries as well as the development of formalized nursing education. Better trained nurses were needed for supervision and teaching positions as medicine dictated hospitalized patients. These initiatives were task oriented and physician directed, holding firm to a 'greater good' belief and a call for citizenship. Within hospitals, "the focus was on the problem, the disability, the disease, and the diagnosis, not the person, his family, his needs, his wholeness, or his humanity (Bevis, 1989, p. 39).

Humanistic Existentialism

As Crowell (2017) posits, the shift to humanism and existentialism has often been cited as a cultural movement and not necessarily a philosophy, and yet the significant swing after World War II from community to self has lasted decades. The ideal holds that it is not enough to know natural science and simple truth, but, rather, the imperative is to understand the whole individual: mind, body, and spirit. If you consider the philosophical periods prior to the humanistic existential period, in which one extreme to the other was valued, this is the first time we see a call for balance between philosophies. Society calls for a combination of spiritual, practical, individual, and now human holistic value merged into one. Existentialism, in its most basic form, can be defined as the acceptance of the individual views of each person, and that reality is defined within each person's mind. Reality is what we individually say it is, and we are each responsible for our own destiny and should be held accountable for our own choices (Crowell, 2017). Humanism, on the other hand, stresses the goodness of people and looks to our human needs to solve problems realistically. By definition, it is a way of thinking in which individual human interest prevails. People are accountable for their own choices and are guided by ethics and morality, and yet they are also allowed to search for their own meaning. In this combined view, the attainment of a good life is what we each choose for ourselves and will occur through the intersection of the mind, body, and spirit. This is the first time in history that nurses use the term "holistic" to describe the ideology of nursing and the care provided to people. This combination of individualism, accountability, and holistic human consideration also sparked an entire psychological movement, or what is termed the "me" era in psychology. At the beginning of this philosophical period, nursing sees the development of significant advancement in nursing theory related to humanistic care and holds precious the entitlement to individualized care, the nurse–client relationship, and nursing's autonomy and professional accountability. It is at this crossroads in nursing history that we see evidence of the development of nursing both as an art and as a science. Even today, society holds on to humanistic existentialism as a predominant societal philosophy. Over the last fifty years in the United States, there has been an increasing extreme shift within existential society. This shift has brought about the cultural norms of extreme personal entitlement and a strong focus away from citizenship and community toward "you do you" and "what's in it for me" mentalities. Although the literature defines current philosophy to be once again 'at a turning point,' there is no doubt that societal values, given current world events, will not shift once again to form a new world view.

Select Predominant Nurses in American History

Martha Ballard (1735–1812)

Martha Ballard was a resident of colonial Maine and a well-known midwife and healer of her time. She lived and died before Florence Nightingale was even born, but Martha Ballard's diary still survives. Entitled *A Midwife's Tale*, this book chronicled four years of her life and contains a remarkable record of the lives of pioneer women and the practice of midwifery during the earliest years of the United States, including the Revolutionary War. Martha Ballard was a self-educated nurse, having had no formal training and using only evidence and experience to guide her practice. During her lifetime, she saw the beginning of modern American medicine and kept careful notes of herbs and remedies and their intended or adverse effects. In 1998, PBS created a documentary based on the diary of Martha Ballard, which can be watched for free if you have a membership with Netflix or Amazon Prime Video. For further information, including access to her original diary, go to https://www.pbs.org/wgbh/americanexperience/films/midwife/#film_description.

The Use of the Hippocrates' Four Humors

In the colonial period, care for the sick reflected the contemporary knowledge of health and disease and the methods of care customary in Western Europe. That knowledge had been developed during the renaissance (1300–1600 AD) and was based on the rediscovery of the ancient works of Galen, Hippocrates, and Aristotle from the Ascetic period. During the romantic period, many based healthcare on myth and superstition, which

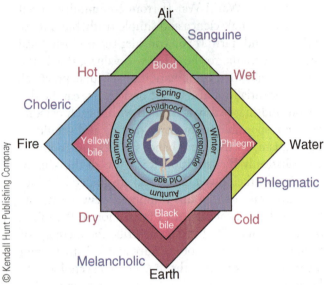

is highlighted in Hippocrates' "the four humors." The four humors from Hippocrates involved the balance of the four elements—fire, air, earth, and water—as evidenced in the four cardinal fluids—yellow bile (fire), blood (air), black bile (earth), and phlegm (water). Illness was an imbalance of the elements and became tied to virtue and religion and food and herbs ("some food brought on good humors, and others, evil humors." A common treatment for leprosy was a "broth made of the flesh of a black snake" (NIH, U.S. National Library of Medicine, 2013).

Throughout the colonial period in the United States, care of the sick was delivered in the home. Many citizens, however, particularly the poor and infirm did not have families to care for them. Almshouses were established to house, feed, and care for the poor. Watch the following video. Did you know that there is still an almshouse in existence? This almshouse still exists in Croydon, England—https://youtu.be/uJIUPJzUT1Q. Whereas the almshouses remaining today are still considered benevolent institutions, the original almshouse was often crowded and filthy and lacked adequate and nutritious food. Poor conditions and the inability to properly treat patients in almshouses would eventually lead to the establishment of the Pennsylvania Hospital in the United States and the Public Hospital for Persons of Insane and Disordered Minds in the mid-18th century.

Dorothea Dix (1802–1887)

In 1841, Dorothea Dix became known as a prominent mental health nurse. As a woman and a stark activist in a time of clearly defined gender roles, she advocated for patients suffering from mental illness by inspecting institutions for signs of mistreatment and working to improve mental health facility conditions. Dorothea Dix was appointed the first woman Superintendent of Army Nurses, creating high nursing standards and working tirelessly to recruit nurses for the Union during the Civil War. During her life, Dorthea Dix fought for better education and training for nurses across the United States and more opportunities for nurses in health care (Norwood, 2017). For more information on Dorothea Dix and mental health reform, see the following video: https://youtu.be/FmkX9s9EH1Q.

Mary Seacole (1805–1881)

In 1857, Mary Seacole, a biracial nurse who served alongside Florence Nightingale during the Crimean War, published her autobiography, *The Wonderful Adventures of Mrs. Seacole in Many Lands*. Mary Seacole, who was born in Jamaica to a Scottish father and Jamaican mother, learned nursing from observing her mother, who often cared for those in a family-owned boarding house in Kingston. Extremely intelligent and resourceful, Mary Seacole traveled around the Caribbean, learning English medical techniques, and eventually traveled to England with the sole intention of joining the Army as a nurse for the Crimean War. Although rejected, Seacole traveled on her own to Crimea, and, as her mother had done, established a hotel specifically to recover wounded officers from the battlefield. Mary Seacole often visited the battlefield itself to provide care to the wounded. At the end of the war, she returned to England and published her autobiography (British Broadcasting Corporation, 2014). For more information on the life of Mary Seacole, watch the short, three-part video series on her life from BBC at: https://www.bbc.co.uk/teach/school-radio/history-ks2-mary-seacole-video/zbphxyc.

Mother Bickerdyke (1817–1901)

Mary Ann Bickerdyke, born in Ohio, grew up in the homes of various relatives before entering Oberlin College and studying nursing. Marrying a prominent local man, who died 10 years later, Mary Ann Bickerdyke supported herself by running a botanical medical apothecary. When the Civil War began, Mary Ann Bickerdyke aided Union forces by delivering supplies to Union forces and caring for soldiers in makeshift hospitals. Her insistence on proper sanitation and cleaning led her to a strong alliance with the development of the U.S. Sanitary Commission in the 1860s. Under her supervision, and in tandem with the march of General Grant down the Mississippi River, Mary Ann Bickerdyke developed a reputation for tending to the sick and wounded and seeing to their every need. She was notably the only person allowed to move between both General Grant and General Sherman's hospital encampments across 19 battlefields. Dedicated to sanitation, and the care of soldiers, she organized ambulance services and walked abandoned battlefields at night, looking for wounded soldiers, earning the title, "Mother" Bickerdyke. She went on to champion many public health causes for both veterans and the poor. Her devotion to the creation and maintenance of the Salvation Army allowed her to work tirelessly to advocate for the proper care of postwar soldiers and veteran nurses through disability pensions (*Encyclopedia Britannica*, 2019). By accessing the Library of Congress, through the following link, you will be able to view the private letters and papers of Mary Ann Bickerdyke still existing today. https://www.loc.gov/collections/mary-ann-bickerdyke-papers/about-this-collection/.

Walt Whitman (1819–1892)

Most prominently known as a journalist, writer, and poet as well as for her book, *Leaves of Grass,* Walt Whitman was born in New York as the second son of a construction worker. In 1862, Whitman, enjoying a career in journalism, was called to nurse his brother, who, having fought in the battle of Fredericksburg in Virginia during the Civil War, suffered a facial wound and needed care. Walt Whitman was very significantly impacted by the suffering of the soldiers and continue to volunteer as a nurse for several years. Without any formal training, Walt Whitman quickly learned from peers and direction from the field doctors, who entrusted him with more and more responsibility. His experience as a nurse influenced his poetry and led to *The Wounded Dresser,* which described his efforts as a Civil War Nurse (AAHN, 2018b). For a short video from PBS on the life of Walt Whitman, see: https://scetv.pbslearningmedia.org/resource/americon-vid-walt-whitman/video/.

Florence Nightingale (1820–1910)

Often heralded as the mother of nursing, Florence Nightingale is equally credited as being the first practicing epidemiologist. In 1860, Florence Nightingale organized the first school of nursing, the *Nightingale Training School for Nurses*, at St. Thomas' Hospital in London, which she modeled after her own philosophy of training. She is well known for improving the sanitation in battlefield hospitals, using her keen mind and statistical analysis to show the connection between poor sanitation and diseases like cholera and dysentery. She kept records of sanitation techniques and became known worldwide as the Lady with the Lamp for her dedication to crossing the battlefields of the Crimean War with her lantern. By improving sanitation in battlefield hospitals, she showed how effective fresh air, hygiene, and nutrition were in the treatment of wounded soldiers, and her methods and care practices remain a basic part of nursing today. For more information on the life of Florence Nightingale, see: https://www.history.com/topics/womens-history/florence-nightingale-1.

Harriet Tubman (1820–1913)

Much is known about the strength and courage of one America's most prominent civil rights activists. Born in Maryland in 1820, as Araminta "Minty" Ross, she was the 11th child of two slaves and endured physical abuse and torture. By her adult life, Harriet, her preferred name, claimed to have spiritual visions, most likely attributed to a serious head trauma sustained by an overseer, which caused headaches, seizures, and vivid dreams, as a child. Harriet Ross went on to marry a free man by the name of John Tubman but continued to remain a slave herself until her escape beyond the border between slaveholding and free states. Harriet Tubman went on to Philadelphia, Pennsylvania, and Maryland, working and saving money. Her mission became bringing family members north, one group at a time, forming what would be known as the Underground Railroad. During the Civil War, Harriet Tubman worked for the Union army as a nurse, a cook, and a spy and, in 1862, moved to Beaufort, South Carolina, while Union occupied, to help the local Sea Island slaves transition to freedom. She eventually moved north and worked in later years to promote civil rights and women's suffrage (Black History in America, 2020). To learn more about Harriet Tubman, see a video special from CBS: https://youtu.be/Ul09jwM9F98.

Clara Barton (1821–1912)

The daughter of a farmer from Massachusetts, Clara Barton, the youngest of five, was first introduced to nursing through her role of caretaker to a chronically ill older brother as a teen. Clara Barton went on to become a teacher, at the insistence of her father, who found her to be too shy and wanted her to resolve her temperament. She founded several schools and later went on to accept a position as the first, ever female government recording clerk at the U.S. Patent office. Both her roles led to her advocacy for equal rights and pay, which fell on deaf ears during multiple presidential administrations. Clara Barton continued, across her entire life, to advocate for women's rights, later joining the women's suffrage movement in the early 1900s. When the Civil War began, Clara Barton made it her mission to bring Union supplies to soldiers and provide disaster relief to people in need. Her work with public aid led to the career and organization she is most well known for today: the creation of the American Red Cross (Michals, 2015). After the civil war, Clara Barton found a new calling that stemmed from the incredible number of families whose family members disappeared during the conflict. Clara Barton attempted to help match soldier data and firsthand accounts with families who were looking for information on a missing loved one. In 1865, she officially created the Missing Soldier's Office, which received more than 60,000 inquires. This office was sanctioned by President Lincoln and went on to publish five separate "Rolls of Missing Men" in newspapers across the country (Clara Barton Missing Soldiers Museum, 2020, para. 1–5). Today, there is a museum dedicated to the Missing Soldiers Office. To learn more about Clara Barton and the Missing Soldiers Office, watch the following video clip: https://youtu.be/M174tKjrUPA.

Mary Mahoney (1845-1926)

In 1878, Mary Mahoney was the first professional black nurse in America. She graduated from the *New England Hospital for Women and Children*, one of the first nursing schools in the United States, after working there as a nurse's assistant, cook, and janitor for 15 years. Following graduation, she continued to work as a private-duty nurse and was readily known for her bedside manner, efficiency, and extreme patience. From an early age, she was concerned with the relationship between cultures and races, which stemmed from attending *The Phillips School* in Boston, one of the first integrated schools in the United States at the time. As a noted nursing leader, Mary Mahoney was among the first to become a member of what became the American Nurses Association. As such, she was one of very few nurses of color among its membership but dedicated her passion and voice as a fierce advocate for race equality and women's rights. Her advocacy led to the cocreation of the National Association of Colored Graduate Nurses (NACGN) and brought forth an awareness of cultural diversity and respect for the individual, regardless of background, race, color, or religion (Spring, 2017a). For more information on the life of Mary Mahoney, see: https://youtu.be/_M4jaCE0LAc.

Linda Richards (1841–1930)

Linda Richards was born in 1841 in New York to devoutly religious parents. Having been witness to the death of both her parents, the care of her wounded fiancé during the Civil War, and influenced by the family doctor, Linda chose a career in nursing. She spent a great deal of time caring for sick neighbors and began her training as an assistant nurse before entering the nursing program newly established by New England Hospital for Women and Children in Boston. She was one of five students accepted into the first class of the program and graduated as the first American trained nurse in 1873. On graduation, Linda Richards became the night supervisor at *Bellevue Hospital Training School* in New York City, which was the first program in the United States to use the Nightingale Model of training. In 1885, after helping to establish nursing schools across the nation, Linda Richards served as a missionary in Japan, where she went on to establish the first Japanese nursing school. She stayed to govern the school for the following five years. On returning to the United States, Linda Richards was extremely active in nursing education and professional organization development and served as the first president of the American Society of Superintendents of Training Schools in 1894. This organization is credited as the very first professional nursing organization in the country (AAHN, 2018a).

Mary Adelaide Nutting (1858–1948)

Considered the first American Professor of Nursing, Mary Nutting was born in 1858 to Canadian parents. Within her studies, she originally trained in the arts and went on to teach music for several years in Newfoundland. In 1889, Johns Hopkins University, in Maryland, announced it was accepting candidates for the first Florence Nightingale nursing training program, and Mary Nutting applied at the age of 31. A two-year program, Mary Nutting graduated in 1891 and was immediately offered employment as head nurse at Johns Hopkins, followed by an appointment in 1892 to assistant superintendent of nurses, superintendent, and, finally, principal of training in 1894. She made several notable changes, including extending the program to three years and adding one of the earliest records of clinical coursework to the nursing curriculum. During this time, Mary Nutting also cofounded the *American Journal of Nursing,* in 1900 and president of the Maryland State Association of Graduated Nurses in 1903 where she created the first nursing practice act in Maryland and became the very first Registered Nurse in the state. In 1906, Mary Adelaide Nutting helped Columbia University, New York, create its first nursing program and accepted a position as its first nursing professor. Notably, she was instrumental in moving nursing education into universities for decades. As nursing education developed, nursing practice also expanded, championing formal education for nurses in the Army and the title of president of the Florence Nightingale International Foundation in 1934. Her many books and impact on nursing led to several national nursing awards, and her many contributions revolutionized professional nursing education, making it what it is today (Spring, 2017b).

Lystra Gretter (1858–1951)

Lystra Eggert-Gretter was born in Ontario, Canada, in 1858 to a Swiss physician and Dutch mother. Thought to have inherited her call to nursing from her mother's dedication to Christian care, Lystra watched as her father enlisted as a surgeon during the American Civil War and subsequently moved with her family to North Carolina, where she studied at private schools. When she was 19 years old, she met and married a Civil War veteran and deputy U.S. marshall. When her husband died, Lystra Gretter was only 26 and, as a single mother, returned to school and attended the Ferrand Training School for Nurses at Harper Hospital in Detroit, Michigan. Graduating with honors in 1888, she was appointed nursing school superintendent, a position she held for many years. Her contributions to nursing are numerous, including lobbying for shorter working hours and an extension to nursing education training programs from one to three years; the recruitment of nurses for the Daughters of the American revolution Hospital Corp during the Spanish American War; the creation of the Detroit Visiting Nurses Association; and the first elected president of the Michigan Nurses Association. Her most famous contribution, however, was the creation of the original Nightingale Pledge. An adaptation of the Hippocratic Oath taken by physicians, the Nightingale Pledge remains one of the most symbolic nursing pledges recited to this day by American nurses at graduation:

> ~~~I solemnly pledge myself, before God and in the presence of this assembly, to pass my life in purity and to practice my profession faithfully. I will abstain from whatever is deleterious and mischievous and will not take or knowingly administer any harmful drug. I will do all in my power to maintain and elevate the standard of my profession and will hold in confidence all personal matters committed to my keeping and all family affairs coming to my knowledge in the practice of my calling. With loyalty will I endeavor to aid the physician, in his work, and devote myself to the welfare of those committed to my care. ~~~

According to Yates (2020), "Gretter is believed to have written the first standardized textbook for nursing training. She also formed a professional library and encouraged students to remain current in the latest nursing procedures" (Professional Entry: The Farrand Training School for Nurses, para 5). In the advancement of the profession of nursing, Gretter's work in nursing education led to the requirement of a professional license of nurses in Michigan.

Jane Delano (1862–1919)

Most well known as the founder of the American Red Cross Nursing Service, a branch of the American Red Cross begun by Clara Barton, Jane Arminda Delano was born in 1862 in New York after the death of her father from yellow fever in the Union Army during the Civil War. She moved to New York City in 1884 to attend the Bellevue Hospital Training School for Nurses and graduated in 1886. Jane Delano went on to become the superintendent of nurses at Sandhills Hospital in Jacksonville, Florida, a role she specifically chose given her interest in caring for patients with yellow fever. Because of her keen observations, Jane Delano was one of the first to pioneer the use of mosquito nets over patient windows despite mosquitos having not yet been scientifically proven as a source of the disease. She moved on to Arizona to care for patients during the typhoid epidemic and returned to the north in 1891, leading many nursing programs, including Bellevue in 1902. In 1909, she served as president of the Board of Directors of the *American Journal of Nursing*, chairman of the American Red Cross, and was appointed superintendent of the Army Nurse Corp. She is known as the creator of the American Red Cross Nursing Service and established the service as the reserve corps for the Army, Navy, and Public Health Service. Her training programs for nurses assisted many in their recovery from several epidemics during her lifetime, including the deadly influenza pandemic of 1918. She cowrote a textbook and traveled extensively around the world, recruiting women to train nurses and volunteer in the Army (Alexander, 2019). For a short video clip on the life and contributions of Jane Delano, see: https://youtu.be/WrTXy3UmFr4.

Lillian Wald (1867–1940) and Mary Maud Brewster (1864–1901)

Nursing in the community increased significantly in 1893, when Lillian Wald enlisted the support of Mary Brewster, known throughout their lives as passionate educators, nurses, and activists for social welfare, to create and open the Henry Street Settlement. The Henry Street Settlement refers to a physical location in the Lower East Side of New York, which, at the time, comprised several blocks of buildings, or tenements, overflowing with the poorest of New York classes. Both were born to wealthy families and, influenced by the work of Florence Nightingale, chose a life of simple existence to care for the poor in New York City. Lillian Wald and Mary Brewster began a mission of community servanthood in their late 20s, tending to people without judgment, educating them on common basic health practices, providing nutrition assistance, and caring for the gravely ill who had no income. The role of the "public health nurse," a role coined by Lillian Wald, was that of one who visited patients and worked outside of formal health institutions. Both Lillian Wald and Mary Brewster, having graduated together from the New York School of Nursing in 1893, moved to and worked in New York's Lower East Side to bring public health nursing care to tenement housing residents. This revolutionary idea for the poor of New York lent itself heavily to social reform. According to Fee and Bu (2010), "They enrolled six more nurses and several activists, lawyers, union organizers, and social reformers; all lived together and collectively shared living expenses. In addition to nursing, they arranged picnics, excursions to the country, girls' clubs, cooking classes, and tickets to concerts—all in an effort to let their neighbors experience life beyond the tenement and factory" (p. 1206). Still in existence today, these women are credited with the creation of an entire specialty in nursing practice. Their efforts in public health nursing led to the creation of the Visiting Nurse Service of New York, one of the largest nonprofit home care agencies in the world. For more on the beginning of public health nursing and the efforts of Lillian Wald and Mary Brewster, see: https://www.americannursinghistory.org/public-health-nursing.

Additionally, the Henry Street Settlement maintains its own webpage and historical account, which includes a short video, entitled, Baptism By Fire, which can be accessed at https://www.henrystreet.org/about/our-history/exhibit-the-house-on-henry-street/.

Lina Rogers Struthers (1880–1946)

Little is known about Lina Rogers Struthers' life growing up; however, her contributions to nursing and to public health make her one of the most significant nurses in U.S. history. As originally reported by Lina Struthers (1917), in her book, *The School Nurse*, Struthers notes that "on October 1, 1902, Lillian Wald assigned Lina Rogers, a Henry Street Settlement nurse, to promote hygiene and preventive health measures to approximately 10,000 children in four New York City schools as an experiment" (p. 23). In doing so, Lina Struthers became the first school nurse in the United States. The experiment, directed by Lillian Wald, was meant to see what would happen if they embedded a nurse within four public schools in an attempt to improve the health and education of students. At the time, public education was plagued by frequent student illness and absence. According to Hanink (2009), as a consequence of the public health experiment, within 6 months the four schools reported a 90% improvement in student attendance. Documenting every treatment and encounter, Lina Rogers paved the way for the New York City school board to not only fund the addition of nurses to schools but also add more than 400 nurses to schools around New York City. Shortly thereafter, Lina Rogers married a school doctor by the name of William Struthers in 1914. She subsequently went on to replicate her school nursing model in cities across the United States and create a subfield in public health nursing that continues to the present day.

Mary Breckinridge (1881–1965)

Born in 1881, Mary Breckinridge grew up as the daughter of a prominent congressman and U.S. minister to Russia. Because of his role, she traveled extensively as a child, living in Washington, D.C., Russia, and Switzerland before returning to the United States. Mary Breckinridge began training as a nurse at St. Luke's Hospital School of Nursing in New York City and graduated in 1910. After marrying and having two children, both of whom died in 1916 and 1918, respectively, Mary Breckinridge was determined to devote the rest of her life to improving the health of women and children. She briefly took a position with the American Red Cross in France to establish a food and health care program for women and children before later returning to the United States once again to train as a midwife. Breckinridge went on to establish the Frontier Nursing Service, which began in Leslie County, Kentucky, in 1925. The Service was developed as a method to reach and care for the poor, rural, and underserved population in Kentucky. It was the first organization in the United States that used nurses as midwives (*Encyclopedia Britannica*, 2020). For more information on the contributions of Mary Breckinridge, see this real footage and silent film entitled *The Forgotten Frontier*, from the Library of Congress: https://youtu.be/xvNi6wxsiME.

Susie Walking Bear Yellowtail (1903–1981)

Susie Walking Bear Yellowtail became the first American Indian registered nurse and was one of the first of her nation to obtain degrees in higher education. Born in 1903 and later orphaned, Susie Walking Bear grew up in boarding schools on the Crow Reservation until her foster parents sent her to a private Baptist Seminary School in Massachusetts. Susie Walking Bear enrolled in the Boston City Hospital School of Nursing and graduated with honors in 1923. A member of the Crow Indian people, she went on to marry Thomas Yellowtail and care for indigenous people both at the first government-run hospital for the Crow and then within the Public Health Service. Susie Walking Bear Yellowtail championed improvements to the Indian Health Service and created community outreach programs on reservations. Throughout her life, Susie Walking Bear Yellowtail served on Indian Health and education councils and received a special appointment to the President's Council on Indian Education and Nutrition under three different presidents. She advocated for better living conditions, health care, and access. She received the President's Award for Outstanding Nursing Health Care in 1962 under John F. Kennedy (Montana Historical Society, 2014).

Hector Hugo Gonzalez (1937–present)

Born in 1937 in Texas, Hector Hugo Gonzalez, a descendant of original Spaniards who settled Texas in 1750, is credited as one of the first Hispanic American nurses in the United States, co-founder of the National

Association of Hispanic Nurses (NAHN), and the first Mexican American nurse to obtain a PhD. He attended a hospital school for nursing and went on to obtain a bachelor's degree in nursing in San Antonio, TX, followed by a master's degree in Nursing Education and a PhD in Higher Education. Dr. Gonzalez served for two years in the United States Army Corp of Nursing and taught nursing for the Incarnate Word College. He quickly ascended in leadership positions both within the Texas Nurses Association and then as chairman of the Department of Nursing Education at San Antonio College, which is known to be the first two-year nursing program in the country to obtain accreditation from the National League for Nursing with a part-time and full-time evening nursing program for working adults. As cocreator and president of the NAHN, Gonzalez went on to be known as a trailblazer on the board of directors of the National League for Nursing, writing the first position paper on *Nursing's Responsibility to Minorities; see* National League for Nursing Position Statement on nursing's responsibility to minorities and disadvantaged groups. (1979). *NLN publications*, (11-1771), 1–4. His leadership and constant advocacy for minority nursing has reshaped the landscape of modern nursing education (NAHN, 2020).

The foregoing nurses represent only a small proportion of nurses in American history that have made a significant contribution to the advancement of nursing. These nurses, along with many more, including nurses as recent as 2016, have been inducted into the American Association of Nursing Hall of Fame. Their biographies and photos can be accessed using the following link: https://www.nursingworld.org/ana/about-ana/history/hall-of-fame/.

Highlights in the Development of Nursing by Decade

View the following *Timeline of Nursing History*, covering the 17th through 20th centuries at the University of Pennsylvania School of Nursing website: https://www.nursing.upenn.edu/nhhc/nursing-through-time/.

Current Challenges: Nursing in the 21st century

Today, the profession faces multiple challenges. Nurses and nurse educators are revising nursing practice and school curricula to meet the ever-changing needs of society, including an aging population, bioterrorism, emerging infections, and disaster management. Advances in technology and informatics, the high acuity level of care of hospitalized patients, and early discharge from health care institutions require nurses in all settings to have a strong and current knowledge base from which to practice. Nursing organizations and the Robert Wood Johnson Foundation (RWJF) are currently involved in programs to support nursing scholars, decrease the nursing shortage, and improve the health of the nation's population. Nursing is taking a leadership role in developing standards and policies to address the needs of the population now and in the future to include changes in curriculum, advances in technology and informatics, new programs to address emerging health concerns, and a leadership role in developing standards and policies.

In 2000, the regulatory landscape began to shift when Maryland signed into law the first health care compact—the Nurse Licensure Compact (NLC). By 2007, The International Council of Nurses (ICN) held its first global conference in Yokohama, Japan. Comprised of international nursing organizations such as our American Nurses Association, the ICN seeks to set up networking and educational experiences for professional nurses who work all over the world.

By 2008, of the 3,063,163 licensed registered nurses in the United States, only 6.6% were men compared with a near 100% during the Middle Ages.

2010–2020

Our current trends in nursing continue to take shape out of societal need. Nurses throughout history have been quick to respond to and champion new directions in nursing science and hold firm to the notion of humanistic care. In recent years, nursing has witnessed the shift of health care once more out of the hospital and back into outpatient and home settings. With the rise of outbreaks, epidemics, and pandemics, as well as access issues and the escalating cost of health care, new technologies are being engineered to care for patients like never before in the community. Telehealth technology advancement has quickly risen out of the need for social distancing, influenza pandemics, Ebola, Zika, and Covid-19. As of 2021, 34 states will have adopted the NLC, a revision to the more than 100-year-old registration process for RNs. This will allow registered nurses, for the first time in history, to work across state boundaries as nurses keep pace with modern health care delivery (National Council of State Boards of Nursing, 2020). As we have learned from history, changes in society lead to changes in nursing. As we look to the future in professional nursing practice, several trends emerge. There is a renewed focus on the self-care of the nurse. As posited by Jean Watson (2008); we cannot care for others until we learn to wholly care for oneself. As compassion fatigue, secondary traumatic stress, and burnout impact the health and wellness of nurses and the quality of care provided to patients, we look to new strategies to improve resiliency skills to better manage the stressors. Interventions in the health care agency alone are not enough. Nurses need to be self-aware, allowing them to identify effective interventions that help professionals manage health-related risk factors from prolonged caregiver stress.

A second trend in nursing continues to be shaped by the Affordable Care Act of 2010. The ACA affects how health care is paid for and delivered, and nursing envisions that there will be greater emphasis on health promotion, disease prevention, and illness management in the future. More nursing services will be in community-based care settings. As a result, more nurses will be needed to practice in community care centers, schools, and senior centers. This will require nurses to be better able to access resources, identify service gaps, and help patients adapt so as to be able to safely return to their community.

Third, skyrocketing health care costs present challenges to the nursing profession, consumer, and health care delivery system. As a nurse, you are responsible for providing patients with the best-quality care in an efficient and economically sound manner. The issues of unemployment, underemployment, low-paying jobs, mental illness, homelessness, and rising health care costs all contribute to increases in the medically underserved population. In addition, the number of underserved patients who require home-based palliative care services is increasing, and nurses will need to respond to the call.

Over the last ten years, several factors have shape nursing and continue to do so. These factors include evolving technology, genomics, public perception, nursing politics and advocacy, advanced practice roles, population health, disaster and infectious disease training, quality and safety, research, consumerism, health promotion, and the effects of the gender and human rights movements on nursing. The nursing profession will continue to evolve and grow, and so must individual nurses. As we look to you, the next generation of professional nurses, your practice needs to be based on current evidence, not just on your education and experiences and the policies and procedures of health care facilities.

Summary

Why is learning all of this information from nursing history so important? As we move forward, nurses recognize the patterns in history that caused nursing to respond and generate new paths. These reactions, aligned with societal philosophical ideals, will continue to evolve and require nurses to respond with the appropriate innovation, scientific research, and human need response.

References

Alexander, K. L. (2019). *Jane Arminda Delano*. National Women's History Museum. Retrieved from www.womenshistory.org/education-resources/biographies/jane-arminda-delano

American Association for the History of Nursing. (2018a). *Linda A. J. Richards*. Retrieved from https://www.aahn.org/richards

American Association for the History of Nursing. (2018b). *Walt Whitman*. Retrieved from https://www.aahn.org/whitman

British Broadcasting Corporation. (2014). History: Mary Seacole. Retrieved from http://www.bbc.co.uk/history/historic_figures/seacole_mary.shtml

Bevis, E. O. (1989). *Curriculum building in nursing: A process* (3rd ed.). New York, NY: National League for Nursing.

Black History in America. (2020). *Harriet Tubman*. Retrieved from http://www.myblackhistory.net/Harriet_Tubman.htm

Chaska, N. (1990). *The nursing profession: Turning points*. St. Louis, MO: C. V. Mosby.

Clara Barton Missing Soldiers Museum. (2020). *Clara Barton's missing soldiers office*. Retrieved from https://www.clarabartonmuseum.org/mso-short/

Crowell, S. (2017). Existentialism. *The Stanford encyclopedia of philosophy*. Retrieved from https://plato.stanford.edu/archives/win2017/entries/existentialism/

Dock, L. L., & Stewart, I. S. (1938). *A short history of nursing*. New York, NY: G. P. Putnam's.

Encyclopedia Britannica. (2019). Mary Ann Bickerdyke. Retrieved from https://www.britannica.com/biography/Mary-Ann-Bickerdyke

Encyclopedia Britannica. (2020). Mary Breckinridge. Retrieved from https://www.britannica.com/biography/Mary-Breckinridge

Fee, E., & Bu, L. (2010). The origins of public health nursing: The Henry Street Visiting Nurse Service. *American Journal of Public Health*, *100*(7), 1206–1207. Retrieved from https://doi.org/10.2105/AJPH.2009.186049

Hanink, E. (2009). Lina Rogers, the First School Nurse: Spearheading an intervention to keep kids in school. *Working Nurse*. Retrieved from http://www.workingnurse.com/articles/lina-rogers-the-first-school-nurse

Merriam-Webster Dictionary. (2020). Bedlam [definition]. Retrieved from https://www.merriam-webster.com/dictionary/bedlam

Michals, D. (2015). *Clara Barton*. National Women's History Museum. Retrieved from https://www.womenshistory.org/education-resources/biographies/clara-barton

Montana Historical Society. (2014). *Susie Walking Bear Yellowtail: "Our bright morning star."* Women's History Matters Biography. Retrieved from http://montanawomenshistory.org/susie-walking-bear-yellowtail-our-bright-morning-star/

National Association of Hispanic Nurses. (2020). *Hector Hugo Gonzalez*. Retrieved from http://nahnnet.org/NAHN/Content/Hector_Hugo_Gonzalez.aspx

National Council of State Boards of Nursing. (2020). NLC fact sheet. Retrieved from https://www.ncsbn.org/NLC_Facts-FINAL.pdf

Norwood, A. R. (2017). Dorothea Dix. Retrieved from https://www.womenshistory.org/education-resources/biographies/dorothea-dix

Spring, K. A. (2017a). *Mary Eliza Mahoney*. Retrieved from https://www.womenshistory.org/education-resources/biographies/mary-mahoney

Spring, K. A. (2017b). *Mary Nutting*. National Women's History Museum. Retrieved from www.womenshistory.org/education-resources/biographies/mary-nutting

Struthers, L. R. (1917). *The school nurse: A survey of the duties and responsibilities of the nurse in maintenance of health and physical perfection and the prevention of disease among school children*. New York, NY: G. P. Putnam.

University of Pennsylvania School of Nursing. (2011). *Nursing, history and health care: Nursing through time*. National Women's History Museum. Retrieved from https://www.nursing.upenn.edu/nhhc/nursing-through-time/

Chapter 3

Professional Nursing

Chapter Objectives:

- Compare and contrast the difference between profession, job, and career
- Describe the characteristics of an RN
- Discuss the value of professional nursing organizations
- Define the ethical principles of nursing and the student nurse
- Describe the ethical theories used in health care
- Describe the nursing role in ethical practice
- Define an ethical dilemma
- Discuss current ethical issues in health care

What does it mean to be a nurse? We have reviewed nursing roles and the implications of nursing history, and yet sometimes what we read in a text seems more theoretical than tangible. Yet the sheer scope of nursing cannot be fully comprehended without knowing from where we came and how we evolved, not just for others but for ourselves. The image that many people hold in their minds of a nurse can often be difficult to describe because they base that description on real experience and everyday encounters. In nursing, the ideals of a profession prove far more significant emotionally than perhaps other fields, not because of a uniform sense of politeness but rather because of nursing's dedication to honoring the values of respect, advocacy, and responsibility associated with a true focus on individual holistic care coming before all else.

Take a moment now to watch *What if You Became a Nurse*, by Sana Goldberg: https://youtu.be/0WnLA6bSmwA and reflect on the complexity of what nursing is and what it means in society.

Profession versus Job versus Career

Although many people casually use the terms "profession/al," "job," and "career" interchangeably, you may have never stopped to consider the difference. Often, when images of a professional come to mind, we imagine business attire, briefcases, and perhaps an office building in a big city. Is this really what it means, however, to have a profession or to be a professional? Could you be a professional and not wear business attire or work in a big office building? Absolutely! And yet images of words do shape our impression of roles. So let's investigate this a bit further. A profession, according to *Merriam-Webster* (2020d), is "a calling requiring specialized knowledge and often long and intensive academic preparation."

A true profession is governed by a code of conduct, a guideline for how the discipline will practice, and is regulated by an organization or agency that determines the kind of knowledge and training required. Within a profession, we find very specific educational criteria either in the form of formal higher education or a series of trainings and certifications acknowledging that you have the correct skills and abide by the appropriate standards. Additionally, there are specific characteristics that frame a profession/al that become the core values of

Table 3.1 Characteristics of the Professional Registered Nurse

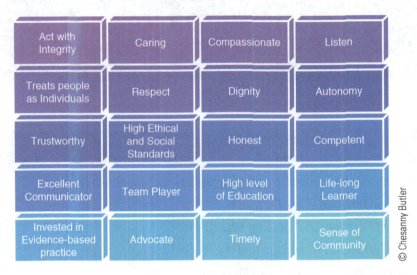

the individuals having the professional credentials. What do you believe are the key characteristics of a professional Registered Nurse? Table 3.1 presents the characteristics of a professional RN.

How is a profession different than a job? Although no single factor can absolutely differentiate a job from a profession, the caveat is how you choose to practice. To act professionally, you provide high-quality patient-centered care in a safe, prudent, and knowledgeable manner. You become immediately accountable for your actions and those of your peers as well as the life of your patient.

Think for a moment about a past employment opportunity. When we talk about a job, most of us think about a position in a company that we took for a brief period of time. Perhaps we did not love the employment opportunity, but we tried to find a position that would (1) align with what we thought we could do and (2) provided us with an income. Maybe we were exploring different kinds of opportunities to see if we enjoyed a specific industry, or, perhaps, we were taking the position out of necessity. A job, as defined by *Merriam-Webster* (2020b), is simply "something done for private advantage…a regular remunerative position." Often, we support ourselves, and even our families, by taking numerous jobs throughout our lives to connect the pieces or develop a path to a career that we have had in mind but that requires additional education or training. A career, then, when we think for a moment to ourselves, is something more than a job and yet still different than a profession. A career, as defined by *Merriam-Webster* (2020a), is "a field for or pursuit of consecutive progressive achievement especially in public, professional, or business life." It often involves the term "profession," and yet it refers to a span of time, often a lifetime, in which a person undertakes the various requirements as a permanent calling. Although similar, there are key differences between a career and a profession. First, while a profession can be understood to be a type of occupation that requires extensive training, perhaps licensure and certification or consecutive educational degrees, a career is truly that sequence of similar jobs from which one gains experience and leads to titles, increasing leadership responsibilities, and accomplishments. Although a profession is an occupation, we can see that a career includes an occupation to the extent that it involves the consecutive roles you have over a lifetime that are organized around a field such as nursing or criminal justice. Third, we know that a profession requires education and that this education and training is constant and continuous to ensure we keep up to date on the ever-changing climate; conversely, a career requires you to have the aspiration and ambition to embrace your profession. This makes a career growth oriented and a profession service oriented, which means we have the knowledge and expertise to provide the service requested to our community. Finally, we understand that as a profession/al, there is a set of rules or some form of guideline framed by a governing or accrediting organization that tells us how we will practice. A career, on the other hand, is not regulated by any set of rules and simply defines the pursuit of employment within a specific field.

When you watch or read the news, chances are you have seen reports of health care advocacy groups working hard to ensure health care consumers find adequate, appropriate, and accessible care. They are also very concerned about the quality of care people receive, not to mention the cost. Consumers of health care often look at reviews of health care providers and facilities online before deciding to use their services. Nursing recognizes that people must become part of the health care team and that they need to be able to trust the care they receive. Nursing values the importance that the role of professional nursing has on health care in the United States. The Robert Wood Johnson Foundation (RWJF) *Future of Nursing: Campaign for Action* (RWJF, 2014) is a multifaceted campaign designed to transform health care through nursing. Together with the Institute of Medicine's (IOM) publication on *The Future of Nursing: Leading Change, Advancing Health* (IOM, 2010) https://www.ic4n.org/wp-content/uploads/2018/03/The-Future-of-Nursing-Report-2010.pdf, these initiatives prepare professionals in the nursing workforce to meet the health promotion, illness prevention, and complex care needs of the population in our ever-changing health care system.

As students pursuing a nursing degree, you will begin developing and growing your professional practice through numerous clinical as well as scholarly experiences. Your practice as a student nurse will equally be governed by professional organizations, codes of conduct, and a student nurse scope of practice. As a student, it is highly recommended that you begin these professional affiliations upon acceptance to nursing school to network with and learn from your peers across the country. The professional organization that governs student nurses is called the National Student Nurses Association (NSNA). In addition to this national association, your own school should also have a Student Nurses Association (SNA) that will provide education, resources, experience, advocacy opportunities, and even scholarships. Additionally, talking with your professors about student memberships to national specialty organizations can also be beneficial, especially if you already know what kind of nurse specialty you would like to pursue. More information about the NSNA organization and how you can become a member can be found at: https://www.nsna.org.

Sigma Theta Tau International (STTI) is another student nursing organization that requires an invitation to join. Sigma's mission is to "develop nurse leaders anywhere to improve healthcare everywhere" and is available to BSN and MSN student nurses who have demonstrated exceptional leadership capacity and maintained excellence academically during school. You can find out more about STTI: https://www.sigmanursing.org.

Ethical Responsibilities in Professional Nursing Practice

Although a profession has standards and scopes of practice, they also have an established ethical code to which all members subscribe. Ethics, in general, is the study of conduct and character and is concerned with determining what is good or valuable for individuals, groups, and society at large. Acts that are ethical reflect a commitment to standards that individuals, professions, and societies strive to meet. When decisions must be made about health care, understandable disagreement can occur among health care providers, families, patients, friends, and people in the community, based on a number of influencing factors. The right thing to do can be hard to determine when ethics, values, and perceptions about health care collide. Although you will have extensive ethical training throughout nursing school, here we will describe the basic concepts that will help you embrace the role of ethics in your professional life and promote resolution when an ethical dilemma develops. First, let us review the basic principles or underlying foundation of nursing ethical conduct.

Ethical Principles for Nursing Care	
Autonomy	Commitment to include patients in decisions
Beneficence	Taking positive actions to help others
Nonmaleficence	Avoidance of harm or hurt
Justice	Being fair
Fidelity	Agreement to keep promises
Veracity	A commitment to tell the truth

The foregoing ethical principles for nursing care form the foundation of nursing's professional ethical code. Provided by the American Nurses Association (ANA), the nursing code of ethics, known as the *Code of Ethics for Nurses With Interpretive Statements* (American Nurses Association, 2015), https://www.nursingworld.org/practice-policy/nursing-excellence/ethics/code-of-ethics-for-nurses/coe-view-only/, gives us a guideline and context of practice. Additionally, a global code of ethics has been developed through the International Council of Nurses and is entitled *The ICN Code of Ethics for Nurses* (International Council of Nurses, 2012).

Both documents establish the expectations and ethical standards by which nursing, in the United States and around the world, will be conducted. Before we explore these documents further, let us discuss the basic principles of ethics and the philosophical underpinning or lens through which the profession of nursing provides care. These are important concepts as ethical theories and philosophies affect judgments about what is right and wrong and shape how each of us has created our own viewpoint of the world.

Student Nurse Code of Ethics and Bill of Rights

Did you know that the NSNA has created a code of ethics? This document contains a code of conduct specific to the role of the nursing student in both the academic and clinical settings. Additionally, it houses sections addressing not only a specific code of conduct with specific examples and interpretive statement, but also a nursing student bill of rights, code of professional conduct, and core value statement. Take a look here: https://www.dropbox.com/s/a229ong58d5jx4p/Code%20of%20Ethics.pdf?dl=0.

The intention of the document is to help student nurses not only understand their roles and responsibilities but also help students align with the professional values required in professional nursing practice.

Ethical Theories and Ethical Decision-Making in Nursing

Historically, health care ethics is comprised of a constant search for fixed standards that would determine right action. Ethics has grown into a complex field of study, more flexible than fixed, filled with differences of opinion and deeply meaningful efforts to understand human interaction. These philosophies, or theories on ethics, provide a foundation for developing strategies to use when an ethical dilemma occurs. Ethical theories examine principles, ideas, viewpoints, or philosophies that influence how we make decisions.

Deontology: Defines actions as right or wrong, forms the foundation of nursing practice
Classic Utilitarianism: Proposes that the value of something is determined by its usefulness and provides the greatest good for the greatest number
Feminist Ethics: Focuses on the inequality between people
Bioethics: the practical application of moral consideration in real-world situations
Care Ethics or "Ethics of Care": Emphasizes the importance of understanding relationships, especially as they are revealed in personal narratives

Ethical Dilemmas

An ethical dilemma in nursing is a clinical practice problem that often involves more than one possible choice and is based on the varying values and beliefs of those involved. In order to properly address ethical concerns, nurses must rely on their training in the application of ethical theory and decision-making. It is often a decision that is a balance between scientific evidence and subscribed morality.

Although being involved in an ethical dilemma can be stressful, it is important that you have a clear understanding of some common ethical theories used by nurses worldwide in their provision of care and ethical decision-making.

In facing an ethical dilemma, what steps should the nurse take to begin analyzing the situation?

- First, begin by determining whether the situation is in fact an ethical dilemma. The only way to do this is to gather as much relevant information as possible about the situation in an unbiased fashion.
- Secondly, nurses should pause to reflect on their own values so as not to confuse the issue in question. (We will discuss clarifying value later in this chapter).
- Third, determine medical indications using the principles of beneficence and nonmaleficence.
- Fourth, consider the situation with regard to quality of life using the principle of respect for autonomy.
- Fifth, consider the patient's preferences and capacity for decision-making? Is the patient competent? Is there a legal document indicating preferences for treatment?
- Consider contextual features using the principles of loyalty and fairness on all sides. What is the legal implication? Are there financial, religious, or cultural factors? Are there any conflicts of interest involved?
- Create a pros and cons list, meaning, take the time to list and analyze all possible options in the ethical theory that best fits the situation, the professional standards that are applicable, and the values and beliefs of the patient.
- Finally, work through each theory and apply the decisions to the dilemma so that you can critically analyze the outcome and pick the best decision. Use this process to work with other colleagues.
- Sometimes, the ethical dilemma involves multiple disciplines or may involve a legal concern. In this case, the issue may require a higher-level decision and need to be submitted to an ethics committee.

Source: Jonsen, A. R., Siegler, M., & Winslade, W. J. (2006). *Clinical ethics: A practical approach to ethical decisions in clinical medicine* (6th ed.). New York, NY: McGraw-Hill.

Classic Utilitarianism

Although complex, classic utilitarianism can be simplified to mean that the correct path is the one that offers the greatest good for the largest number involved in the situation. Whereas utilitarianism involves various forms of consequentialism and hedonism, classic utilitarianism, theoretically, has appeal in health care systems. But consider the impact that this theory has on individualism in nursing practice. If a nurse used utilitarianism as a foundation for practice, would we have individualized treatment plans, or would we provide care to everyone in a way that reflected only what was best for the group, not the individual. In this ethical theory, nurses would have to make decisions on your personal care based not on what was best for you and your situation but rather based on what was good for everyone. This could be problematic. Consider the following example: J. Thomas RN is administering medication to the patients on the postsurgical floor. The pharmacy sends every patient the same antibiotic because it is what is most cost effective and efficient in preventing infection after a surgery. You notice that the patient in Room 1 is allergic to the antibiotic. You have a choice: You either can give the patient the medication, knowing that he or she might have an allergic reaction to the medication, or you can hold the medication, increasing that patient's risk for infection. In this ethical theory, you cannot obtain a different antibiotic for one individual patient, despite the reason, because it does not benefit the greatest number of people on the floor. Is this the ethical code that a professional RN should align themselves with for daily practice?

To explore utilitarianism further, see the following from the Stanford Encyclopedia of Philosophy: https://plato.stanford.edu/entries/utilitarianism-history/.

Feminist Ethics

Feminist ethics may be incorrectly labeled because it gives the impression in the naming of the form that this theory involves solely women's rights on the basis of sexual equality. Feminist ethics is, however, so much more complex and inclusive. It critiques conventional ethics such as deontology and utilitarianism and looks to the nature of relationships to guide participants in making difficult decisions, especially relationships in which power is unequal or in which a point of view has become ignored or invisible. Writers with a feminist perspective tend to concentrate more on practical solutions than on theory. Feminist ethicists propose that the natural human urge to be influenced by relationships is a positive value and focuses on power relationships and issues of dominance within nursing practice. For more information on the application of feminist ethics in nursing practice, see Green (2012).

Bioethics

Bioethics is a large category of theories that fall under applied ethics or the practical application of moral consideration in real-world situations. This form of ethics deals with difficult moral questions and controversial moral dilemmas that people face every day.

As defined by Gordon (2020), Bioethics is

> a particular way of ethical reasoning and decision making that: (i) integrates empirical data from relevant natural sciences, most notably medicine in the case of medical ethics, and (ii) considers other disciplines of applied ethics such as research ethics, information ethics, social ethics, feminist ethics, religious ethics, political ethics, and ethics of law in order to solve the case in question (Preliminary distinctions, para 2). https://www.iep.utm.edu/bioethic/.

The Consensus of Bioethics

As you can imagine, there are numerous instances, not in nursing alone, but across the entirety of health care that require a discussion about how patient care might proceed or will be conducted involving difficult moral and ethical decisions. When these types of situations arise, hospitals rely on ethical committees. A hospital ethics committee, or HEC, is comprised of professionals from a number of disciplines who work within a health care setting. These committees often include representatives from medicine, nursing, spiritual and religious services, legal, social work, and other special consultation experts. The value of these committees is significant in that they specifically help providers, and sometimes even patients and their families, deal with ethical challenges raised during a patient's admission and ongoing hospitalization. Their role is specifically to provide ethical case consultation, education, and policy recommendation. Nurses are integral to an ethics committee because they provide insight about ethical problems stemming from their involvement in family conferences, staff meetings, and even in one-on-one interactions with patients. Many ethical problems begin when people feel misled or are not aware of their options and do not know when to speak up about their concerns. Ethics committees serve to complement relationships within the workplace and the community and offer a valuable resource for strengthening these relationships. A process for resolving ethical dilemmas that respects differences of opinion and all participants equally helps health care providers resolve conflict about right actions.

For more information about hospital ethic committee role and involvement, see Hajibabaee, Joolaee, Cheraghi, Salari, and Rodney (2016).

A consensus of bioethics is, therefore, the agreement or majority opinion of the ethics committee and is used as a mechanism to provide their recommendation on the ethical situation presented on the basis of all considerations, values, belief systems, legal aspects, and circumstances in each case.

To learn more information on *The Value of Consensus*, see Chapter 14 of *Society's Choices: Social and Ethical Decision Making in Biomedicine* (Benjamin, 1995).

Care Ethics or "Ethics of Care"

Care ethics, also widely known as "the ethics of care," is another ethical theory based on a feminist philosophical foundation that is socially based and focuses on the relationships and dependencies in everyday human life.

Thus, the ethics of care and feminist ethics are closely related. Although we see care ethics purported commonly as a mechanism of practice or a simple ethical virtue (a moral behavior involving high standards), it aligns with nursing's belief that in order to care and meet the needs of others we must also care and meet our own needs. It specifically highlights the personal narrative of the caring relationship. The difference is that the ethics of care is based solely on the reciprocity of this relationship as well as the recipient of care's point of view, expectations, and needs. What we find is that this ethical theory is not specifically always applicable to nursing care because the care being requested may not necessarily be rational, based on evidence, live up to patient expectations, or improve a patient's condition. The ethics of care exists in contrast to the liberal platform of equitable justice, but is commonly seen in personal care practice such as end of life care.

To learn more about Care Ethics, see Ethics and Philosophy (Dunn, 2020).

Deontology

In considering whether something is acceptable or not, nursing subscribes to deontological principles. In its simplest form, deontology means that something is either correct or incorrect. The nurse either did something appropriately or correctly or didn't. Deontology depends on a mutual understanding of justice, autonomy, and goodness but leaves little room for causational error because nursing practice involves the care of people. Here is an example: J. Thomas, RN, has an order to administer an antibiotic to the patient in Room 1. She gets distracted and forgets to give the medication. She does not want to get in trouble, so she charts that she gave the patient the medication even though she didn't. Using the principles of deontology, is this situation right or wrong? Does it matter if J. Thomas, RN, had a reason for not giving the medication? What about her ethical conduct or morality in this situation? Is there something wrong in the way the nurse behaves that is unacceptable to professional practice? Deontology defines actions as right or wrong on the basis of their "right-making characteristics," such as fidelity to promises, truthfulness, and justice.

To explore Deontology further, see the following from the Stanford Encyclopedia of Philosophy: https://plato.stanford.edu/entries/ethics-deontological/.

Definitions, Digging Deeper

By definition, a value reflects a personal belief about the worth of a given idea, attitude, custom, or object that sets standards that influence personal morality. Something that we value may be education or honesty. According to *Merriam-Webster* (2020e), a value is "something (such as a principle or quality) intrinsically desired." Ethical dilemmas almost always occur in the presence of conflicting values. To resolve ethical dilemmas, one needs to distinguish among values, facts, and opinion. In most other intimate relationships, you choose to enter the relationship precisely because you anticipate that your values will be shared with the other person. But as a nurse, you agree to provide care to your patients solely on the basis of their need for your services. As a nurse, you will need to respect your own values even as you try to respect those of others whose values differ from yours. To negotiate differences of value, it is important to be clear about your own values: what you value, why, and how you respect your own values even as you try to respect those of others whose values differ from yours. The values that each individual may hold reflect cultural and social influences, and these values vary among people and develop over time.

It is worth noting that people have such strong values that they consider them to be facts, not just opinion. Sometimes, people are so passionate about their values that they become judgmental in a way that intensifies conflict.

Clarifying values—your own, your patients', your coworkers'—is an important and effective part of ethical discourse. In the process of values clarification, you learn to tolerate differences in a way that often (although not always) becomes the key to the resolution of ethical dilemmas. Identifying values as something separate from facts can help you find tolerance for others, even when differences among you seem worlds apart.

Values form together to develop a specific set of behaviors or our expression of morality. A moral or morality specifically reflects personal values and beliefs and directs not only personal behavior or conduct but also decision-making. *Merriam-Webster* (2020c) defines moral as "of or relating to principles of right and wrong in behavior." In comparison, morals or morality are usually interpreted as a personal preference in how we conduct ourselves and are comprised of values; ethics are broader and are equated with a category or overall universality of fairness.

Issues in Health Care Ethics

Quality of life: Central to discussions about end-of-life care, cancer therapy, physician-assisted suicide, and Do Not Resuscitate (DNR)	
Disabilities: Antidiscrimination laws enhance the economic security of people with physical, mental, or emotional challenges	
Care at the end of life: Interventions unlikely to produce benefit for the patient	
Health Care Reform: Facilitated access to care for millions of uninsured Americans	

Ethical issues change as society and technologies change, but common denominators remain: the basic process used to address the issues and your responsibility to deal with them.

These professional ethical/bioethical issues will influence you and the care you give your patients: quality of life, genetic screening, and care at the end of life.

Quality-of-life measures may take into account the age of a patient, the patient's ability to live independently, his or her ability to contribute to society in a gainful way, and other nuanced measures of quality.

Still, a definition remains deeply individual and difficult to predict. The question of quality of life is central to discussions about quality of care, outcome measures, care at the end of life, futile care, cancer therapy, and health care provider–assisted suicide. The national movement to respect the abilities of all, regardless of their functional status, has inspired a reconsideration of the definition of quality of life. Antidiscrimination laws enhance the economic security of people with physical, mental, or emotional challenges.

The *capabilities approach* begins with a commitment to the equal dignity of all people, whatever their class, religion, caste, race, or gender, and it is committed to the attainment, for all, of lives that are worthy of that equal dignity.

Difficult emotional and spiritual challenges resulting in moral distress can characterize the management of care at the end of life.

The term *futile* refers to something that is hopeless or serves no useful purpose. In health care discussions, the term refers to interventions unlikely to produce benefit for a patient.

If a patient is dying of a condition with little or no hope of recovery, almost any intervention beyond symptom management and comfort measures is seen as futile.

In this situation, an agreement to label an intervention as futile can help providers, families, and patients turn to palliative care measures as a more constructive approach to the situation.

The legislation also incorporates a promotion of wellness by proposing changes in payment for services and by rewarding practices that reduce harm and promote quality outcomes.

The American Nurses Association Code of Ethics

In nursing, the basic principles of responsibility, accountability, advocacy, and confidentiality remain constant and are a focus of the ANA's Code of Ethics. Advocacy refers to the support of a particular cause. As a nurse, you advocate for the health, safety, and rights of patients, including their right to privacy and their right to refuse treatment. Responsibility refers to willingness to respect obligations and to follow through on promises. Accountability refers to the ability to answer for one's own actions. Another critical component of nursing

Provisions of the Code of Ethics for Nurses with Interpretive Statements	
Provision 1	The nurse practices with compassion and respect for the inherent dignity, worth, and unique attributes of every person.
Provision 2	The nurse's primary commitment is to the patient, whether an individual, family, group, community, or population
Provision 3	The nurse promotes, advocates for, and protects the rights, health, and safety of the patient
Provision 4	The nurse has authority, accountability, and responsibility for nursing practice; makes decisions; and takes action consistent with the obligation to promote health and to provide optimal care
Provision 5	The nurse owes the same duties to self as to others, including the responsibility to promote health and safety, preserve wholeness of character and integrity, maintain competence, and continue personal and professional growth
Provision 6	The nurse, through individual and collective effort, establishes, maintains, and improves the ethical environment of the work setting and conditions of employment that are conducive to safe, quality health care
Provision 7	The nurse, in all roles and settings, advances the profession through research and scholarly inquiry, professional standards development, and the generation of both nursing and health policy
Provision 8	The nurse collaborates with other health professionals and the public to protect human rights, promote health diplomacy, and reduce health disparities
Provision 9	The profession of nursing, collectively through its professional organizations, must articulate nursing values, maintain the integrity of the profession, and integrate principles of social justice into nursing and health policy

Source: American Nurses Association (2015). Used by permission.

ethics involves the concept of confidentiality. When we talk about the importance of confidentiality, we are talking about protecting information that is held in confidence with very specific groups of people such as doctors, nurses, and lawyers. Confidential information is based on the "need to know" in order to properly care for an individual and is not available to any other member unless he or she is directly involved in the care of the patient. Conversely, privacy, which is often used synonymously with confidentiality, "refers to the freedom from intrusion into one's personal matters, and personal information. We often use the terms 'confidentiality' and 'privacy' interchangeably in our everyday lives. However, they mean distinctly different things from a legal standpoint" (FindLaw, 2020, para 1).

Confidential information can also not be shared without the written consent of the patient involved. This can mean that information about a patient's health, prognosis, or treatment can often not be legally shared with immediate family members unless the patient has given clinicians permission to include those specific people in their care. Because of the complexity and seriousness of confidentiality, health care facilities have compliance officers who are responsible for making sure that the institution remains in compliance with standards and regulations. One of the most significant pieces of legislation with regard to confidentiality includes the Health Insurance Portability and Accountability Act of 1996 (HIPAA), which mandates the protection of a patient's personal health information. In recent years, nursing and health care have been challenged with new ethical dilemmas surrounding confidential information and the use of technology. Social networks can be a supportive source of information about patient care or professional nursing activities and can also be a significant risk to patient privacy. Because of this, the ANA and the NSNA have developed guidelines and tips for the use of technology and social media in the practice environment.

See the ANA's Principles for Social Networking and the Nurse: https://www.nursingworld.org/~4af4f2/globalassets/docs/ana/ethics/social-networking.pdf

See the Image of Nursing Committee's NSNA Social Media Tips Do's and Don'ts: https://www.dropbox.com/s/vvku9nbv407ei61/NSNA%20Social%20Media%20Tips.pdf?dl=0

Consider the student who is so excited to have witnessed their very first birth, while attending clinical, on a labor and delivery unit. The student can't wait to post a picture of the baby that they took in the nursery and tell their family all about the amazing clinical experience. It wouldn't be a problem if the student posted the photo as long as it didn't contain a way to identify the baby or the family…right…? Wrong! Sometimes, the patient can still be identified by family, friends, or other health care workers because of the location or significance of the event. Sometimes, the description, the photo, or both are reposted because others liked the story or wanted to share how proud they are of the student nurse. In addition to professional practice guidelines, students and nurses must also adhere to workplace policies because they help guide decisions while engaging patients and determining proper ethical behavior.

Summary

In this chapter, the critical differences between a profession, job, and career were identified as learners discovered nursing as a professional science. The characteristics of a professional nurse were explored, and the values of professional nursing organizations were discussed, helping to clarify the standards of practice and ethical principles that form the fabric of who and what nurses represent. Multiple ethical theories were identified, and examples of ethical dilemmas brought forth the extreme challenges faced by health care teams in daily practice. As the role of the RN was clarified in ethical conduct and care, the use of bioethics and ethic committees centralized the need for team approaches to patient safety and care.

References

American Nurses Association. (2015). Code of ethics for nurses with interpretive statements. Silver Spring, MD: Author. Retrieved from https://www.nursingworld.org/practice-policy/nursing-excellence/ethics/code-of-ethics-for-nurses/coe-view-only/

Beauchamp, T., & Childress, J. (2012). *Principles of biomedical ethics* (7th ed.). New York, NY: Oxford University Press.

Benjamin, M. (1995). The value of consensus. In R. E. Bulger, E. M. Bobby, & H. V. Fineberg (Eds.), *Society's choices: Social and ethical decision making in biomedicine* (pp. 241–260). Washington, DC: National Academy Press. Retrieved from https://www.nap.edu/read/4771/chapter/14

Dunn, C. P. (2020). Ethics of care. *Encyclopaedia Britannica*. Retrieved from https://www.britannica.com/topic/ethics-of-care

FindLaw. (2020). Is there a difference between confidentiality and privacy? Retrieved from https://criminal.findlaw.com/criminal-rights/is-there-a-difference-between-confidentiality-and-privacy.html

Gordon, J. S. (2020). Bioethics. *Internet encyclopedia of philosophy: A peer-reviewed academic resource*. Retrieved from https://www.iep.utm.edu/bioethic/

Green, B. (2012). Applying feminist ethics of care to nursing practice. *Journal of Nursing & Care, 1*(3), 1–4. doi:10.4172/2167-1168.1000111; Retrieved from https://www.hilarispublisher.com/open-access/applying-feminist-ethics-of-care-to-nursing-practice-2167-1168.1000111.pdf

Hajibabaee, F., Joolaee, S., Cheraghi, M. A., Salari, P., & Rodney, P. (2016). Hospital/clinical ethics committees' notion: An overview. *Journal of Medical Ethics and History of Medicine, 9*, 17. Retrieved from https://www.ncbi.nlm.nih.gov/pmc/articles/PMC5432947/

International Council of Nurses. (2012). The ICN code of ethics for nurses. Retrieved from https://www.icn.ch/sites/default/files/inline-files/2012_ICN_Codeofethicsfornurses_%20eng.pdf

Merriam-Webster Dictionary. (2020a). Career [definition]. Retrieved from https://www.merriam-webster.com/dictionary/career

Merriam-Webster Dictionary. (2020b). Job [definition]. Retrieved from https://www.merriam-webster.com/dictionary/job

Merriam-Webster Dictionary. (2020c). Moral [definition]. Retrieved from https://www.merriam-webster.com/dictionary/moral

Merriam-Webster Dictionary. (2020d). Profession [definition]. Retrieved from https://www.merriam-webster.com/dictionary/profession

Merriam-Webster Dictionary. (2020e). Value [definition]. Retrieved from https://www.merriam-webster.com/dictionary/value

Robert Wood Johnson Foundation. (2014). Future of Nursing: Campaign for Action. Retrieved from https://www.rwjf.org/en/how-we-work/grants-explorer/featured-programs/future-of-nursing--campaign-for-action.html

Chapter 4

The Art and Science of Nursing

Chapter Objectives:

- Describe the difference between the art and science of nursing
- Discuss how both the art and science of nursing are integral to nursing practice
- Define the nursing process as a framework for clinical practice
- Compare and contrast the nursing process with the scientific process
- Compare clinical judgment and critical thinking
- Identify the essential components of critical thinking in nursing practice
- Define reflection and its value in nursing practice
- Discuss the development of the levels of critical thinking in nursing practice
- Verbalize the importance of each critical thinking educational tool
- Discuss the importance of evidence-based practice in nursing care
- Compare the levels of evidence in nursing research and provide examples of each
- Understand the use of the PICOT format in the development of a clinical research question
- Discuss the rationale for the different forms of research used in the science of nursing

As a professional nurse, your role will be to provide care artfully, with compassion and dignity, respecting each person, family, and group of people holistically and working to improve health with the patient as part of the health team.

Nursing as an Art: The art of nursing refers to core principles of nursing as a profession. When we talk about nursing as an art, we are not referring to a piece of art in the literal sense. The art of nursing means human activity that involves the conceptual form or behaviors associated with demonstrating true altruism in providing care. When we think of art, we think of creativity, ingenuity, a view of the world that allows multiple interpretations and meanings. This is what we mean by "the art of nursing." In this context, we are referring to not only the technical skill and emotional involvement required of nurses but also the history and the holistic, compassionate aesthetic of how care is provided. Interestingly, the art of nursing is something that nurses do leave behind every single day with each patient encounter. The art isn't just the way nursing care is provided; it is also a lasting impression of how nursing and care is received. Nursing as an art refers to the impact left behind, forever imprinted in the minds and within the hearts of those we touch. These values are held with extreme regard and include the foundation of care, compassion for others, and highly effective communication. The art of nursing is full of emotion, creativity, ingenuity, human capacity, caring, and compassion. In order to understand nursing as an art, we must take a closer look at some of the discipline's basic artful tenets.

Ways of Caring

Caring, as a central concept, has led to many attempts to explain why we often see the words "care" and "nurse" synonymously (McCance, McKenna, & Boore, 1999). In order to fully understand the ways in which nurses "provide care" and "are caring," we need to dive into theory. First, let's understand that care exists not only as a noun, but also as a verb and an adjective in the field of nursing. Note these differences used in brief sentences: I can "provide care," I can "be caring," and "I care." These distinctions hold explicit meaning in what we know caring to be and the actions associated with caring behaviors. Let's look a bit deeper as the ways we understand caring to be described.

In the 1970s, Leininger's Theory of Cultural Care and Jean Watson's Theory of Human Caring gave rise to the full meaning of nursing care. Madeleine Leininger subscribed to the central tenet that "care is the essence of nursing and the central, dominant, and unifying focus of nursing" (Leininger, 1991) and that this is a universal and global right steeped in culture. According to Leininger (2008):

> Culturally based care factors are recognized as major influences upon human expressions related to health, illness, wellbeing, or to face death and disabilities. Human care is what makes people human, gives dignity to humans, and inspires people to get well and to help others and further predicts there can be no curing without caring, but caring can exist without curing. Care cannot be separated from culture and provides context to health. Culture *and* care together are predicted to be powerful theoretical constructs essential to human health, wellbeing, and survival. In-depth knowledge of the specific culture care values, beliefs, and lifeways of human beings within life's experiences is held as important to unlock a wealth of new knowledge for nursing and health practices (pp. 1–2). http://www.madeleine-leininger.com/cc/overview.pdf

Dr. Jean Watson is another theorist in nursing that has dedicated her life to defining, explaining, and expanding the art of caring in nursing. We will discuss nursing theory in Chapter 5. First, we must look at some basic tenets of how nurses are caring (adjective) so that they can appreciate and learn, more fully, how to provide care (verb).

In Watson (2008, p. 34), six core principles form the foundation of "being caring":

1. Caring for others can begin only when we start by demonstrating care for ourselves and attending to our own well-being. Being mindful and having mindfulness is a concept of maintaining balance in our lives: reducing stress, maintaining psychological and physical wellness, and eliminating burnout. When we care for ourselves, we are better able to provide care through a loving and kind expression to those around us. Caring fully for ourselves allows us to radiate care to others.
2. The second core principle is ensuring that each and every encounter with another is authentic. What does it mean to be present with another person authentically? It means that we are genuine with people, that we are "emotionally appropriate, significant, purposive, and responsible mode of human life" (*Merriam-Webster*, 2020).
3. Third, we must be willing and able to know ourselves well enough so as to be able to identify our own spiritual, mental, and physical needs so that we can move beyond ourselves and meet people where they are in their lives. This means that we are comfortable enough in our own skin, we have accepted ourselves wholly, and we can move past our own egos and not focus on or compare our lives, our beliefs, and our needs and desires with those around us. When we are young adults, it is very difficult sometimes to really know who we are and what we stand for completely. This third core principle takes time, guidance, and practice, but it is acknowledging our path to becoming whole that we can work hard to make every situation about others and not ourselves.
4. The fourth principle in the ways of caring involves being able to develop and sustain relationships. This involves developing trust and cultivating the trusting relationship in a sustainable way that demonstrates love and compassion.
5. Often, we hear people talk about the environment around them. Environment, however, means more than a physical location; it means an atmosphere or a vibe. A nurse imbues care. This means we become the

caring environment because it is present in everything we do, see, say, touch. We are the caring–healing environment genuinely, and people can "read" this about our personality.

6. Finally, the ways of caring involve having an open mind. Many nurses call this being receptive to considering new or different ideas. We serve others in a way that allows for all possibilities, both expected outcomes and inexplicable life events that we may not be able to rationally explain. We allow for the possibilities of miracles and support people in their beliefs. We advocate, we educate, and we allow people to decide for themselves what is best.

No matter how busy or how technical or complex a situation may be, nurses pause, center themselves, and then engage others to ensure that they are listening, seeing, providing touch and care to all patients. Nurses take time to ensure patients are aware that they have value and meaning and that they will be met wherever they are mentally, physically, and/or spiritually. Nurses practice care as an art because it truly takes skill. Nurses have the ability to develop individual plans of care using standards of practice but they do it in a way that demonstrates compassion and authenticity. In a comprehensive literature review, Venes (2020) identifies the top caring behaviors of nurses: Nurses genuinely smile; they communicate and answer questions timely and effectively; they provide hope, make eye contact, use emotional intelligence; they demonstrate respect through action and maintain appropriate personal space; they listen attentively; they provide appropriate therapeutic touch; and, above all, they are compassionate and provide patients with the ability to make their own informed decisions. Hope is guided by our commitment as nurses to our patients. When we talk about providing hope, as mentioned previously, we are describing "an awareness of the moment, alive with possibilities;" nurses honor optimism and fully understand the role that the mind plays in human recovery and well-being (Schoenhofer, 2002, p. 37).

Compassion

We have talked about being "compassionate" in nursing and having "compassion," but what do we know compassion to be? After all, we find these words so commonly used in descriptions of nurses and nursing practice that perhaps we should explore this term and behavior more fully. Compassion is more than kindness. It is more than empathy. It is an artful expression through intentional action expressed and accepted within the nurse–patient relationship. According to the *Merriam-Webster* dictionary (2020), it is "sympathetic consciousness (being aware or having awareness) of others' distress together with a desire to alleviate it." And yet these definitions do not quite seem to capture the entirety of what it means to have compassion in nursing. Published by the Online Greater Good Science Center at University of California at Berkeley (2020),

> Compassion literally means "to suffer together." Among emotion researchers, it is defined as the feeling that arises when you are confronted with another's suffering and feel motivated to relieve that suffering.
>
> Compassion is not the same as empathy or altruism, although the concepts are related. Although empathy refers more generally to our ability to take the perspective of and feel the emotions of another person, compassion is when those feelings and thoughts include the desire to help. Altruism, in turn, is the kind, selfless behavior often prompted by feelings of compassion, although one can feel compassion without acting on it, and altruism isn't always motivated by compassion.

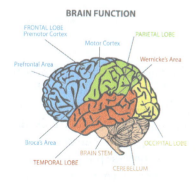

Compassion, therefore, has everything to do with not only a personal feeling and desire but also an experience by a person that the action is intended for. We know that compassion is also not just emotional but deeply biological and results in hormone release for both those providing and those receiving compassion (Keltner, 2009). This hormone, known as oxytocin, along with the right supramarginal gyrus (see image), allows people to want to care for others and provides those receiving the compassion similarly deep emotions.

These physiological responses are responsible for compassion. In a qualitative study by Curtis (2015), three main themes regarding a patient's impression of compassion were noted:

1. patients saw compassion as based on acts that demonstrated human relationships— "knowing me and giving me your time"
2. patients believed the impact of compassion was a sense of empathizing with their situation or "being in their shoes"
3. compassion was the essence of nursing and required communication alongside inherent values-based care (p. 2798).

Compassionate is something that occurs naturally, and yet nursing schools must cultivate compassionate care providers through engagement in environments in which compassionate behaviors are also demonstrated, practiced, and learned.

When nurses combine the art and science of nursing and integrate this into their patient care practice, they significantly increase the quality of care provided to each patient in their care. It is important to know as much about how to care for someone as about how to cure someone. This blend of the art and science of nursing allows us to provide the holistic and individual service that the profession of nursing is known for in society. Having equal strength in both components allows you to provide the best possible care and assures the public that they can trust nurses to always place patients and families first using the most current knowledge and professional practice standards available.

Nursing as a Science: The science of nursing is dependent on systematic knowledge, which needs to be exact and organized. Within all formal science fields, the application of the scientific method is essential. Nursing science requires the same scientific approach not only to patient care but also to research. Within clinical practice, nurses use the nursing process https://www.nursingworld.org/practice-policy/workforce/what-is-nursing/the-nursing-process/, which involves critical thought, clinical judgment, intuition, and perception. Within research, nurses use the scientific method, a highly rigorous endeavor, as a process for creating and performing objective experiments.

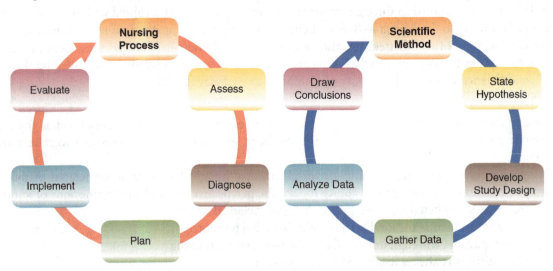

The nursing process is also a framework for practice and can be remembered using the acronym ADPIE. ADPIE stands for the first letter of each step in the process, namely: **A**—Assessment, **D**—Diagnose, **P**—Plan, **I**—Implementation of interventions, **E**—Evaluate. It allows nurses to use overlapping sequential steps that are iterative, not static. This means that the use of the nursing process is ongoing, patient-centered, and ever changing in the pursuit of optimizing care and returning a patient to their fullest capacity for wellness. The nursing process provides a framework through which nurses use knowledge, clinical judgment, critical thought, skill, experience, and standards of practice to shape individual plans of care for each patient.

Torres (1990) shares,

> Basic to any professional discipline is the development of a body of knowledge that can be applied to its practice. Such knowledge is often expressed in terms of concepts and theories, especially in the area of behavioral and social sciences. Thus, nursing as a young, evolving profession is developing a body of knowledge in terms of the concepts and theories that support its practice (p. 1).

Let us pause here, before learning about nursing evidence and research concepts to explore critical thinking and clinical judgment. Understand that both the scientific method and the nursing process require skills, knowledge application, and experience that is nurtured and developed over time. Despite intuitively using thinking skills in our day-to-day activities, we need to focus on the specific components of critical thinking and determine how critical thought is used in nursing practice.

Critical Thinking versus Clinical Judgment

In nursing, critical thinking is the foundation of action. It is defined as the ability to think in a systematic and logic manner with openness to question and reflect on the reasoning process. It requires open-mindedness, continual inquiry, and perseverance combined with a willingness to look at each unique patient situation and determine which of the identified assumptions are true and relevant. This is critical for nurses because a patient's condition can quickly deteriorate. Nurses must be able to quickly recognize a problem, evaluate unfolding information, and draw conclusions that lead to accurate and timely action. Critical thinking is *demonstrated* in nursing by clinical judgment, which includes ethical, diagnostic, and therapeutic dimensions as well as the use of research. Clinical judgment is an essential skill that involves the interpretation of a patient's needs, concerns, or health problems and the decision to take action or not, to use or modify standard approaches, or to improvise new approaches on the basis of a patient's response. Nurses apply knowledge, clinical experiences, and professional standards when thinking critically and making decisions about patient care. As nurses develop professionally, it is important to acquire critical thinking skills that allow you to face each new patient care experience or problem with open-mindedness, creativity, confidence, and continual inquiry.

Essential Components of Critical Thinking

The ability to think critically, improve clinical practice, and decrease errors in clinical judgments is the aim of nursing practice. Learning to apply each element of this model in the way you think about patients will help you become a more confident and effective professional.

Knowledge

Knowledge prepares you to better anticipate and identify patients' problems by understanding their origin and nature. This component requires nurses to embrace lifelong learning and constantly seek to improve their foundational knowledge. As a nurse, your knowledge base includes information and theory from the basic sciences, humanities, behavioral sciences, and nursing. Nurses use their knowledge base in a different way than other health care disciplines because they think holistically about patient problems. The depth and extent of knowledge influence your ability to think critically about nursing problems.

Experience

Clinical learning experiences are necessary to acquire clinical decision–making skills. Has anyone ever told you to gain nursing experience before applying to nursing school? Becoming a nursing assistant or working in another health-related role before applying to nursing school not only helps build foundational knowledge but also gives you experience. Knowledge combined with clinical expertise from experience helps the nurse increase critical thinking. With experience you begin to understand clinical situations, anticipate and recognize cues of patients' health patterns, and interpret the cues as relevant or irrelevant.

Intuition

Experience is what helps develop nursing intuition, or what nurses often call "a red flag." Nurses often sense a problem with a patient developing long before symptoms may appear. This does not happen by accident, and it is not an extra mental gift, like telepathy. Nurses learn to trust intuition as a part of the critical thinking process. This inner sense is fueled by knowledge and experience, which allows the nurse to pause and question why the clinical facts in a case may not align with the clinical picture: perhaps it is a subtle new finding, perhaps it is something stated by the patient. Regardless of how small or insignificant a piece of data may seem, it is intuition or the feeling that drives the nurse with previous experience to recheck and search the data to reconfirm. Nurses use intuition to dig deeper and reflect on relationships between assessment findings and new data and draw new conclusions.

Competency

The nursing process is the general critical thinking scheme or cognitive process that nurses use to develop competency. It is the third component of the critical thinking model. In your nursing practice, you will apply critical thinking components during each step of the nursing process. You will also develop competency in skill and patient care excellence through application of the nursing standards and the incorporation of evidence-based practice into everyday practice.

Attitudes or Mindsets

According to Potter, Griffin-Perry, Stockert, and Hall (2013), there are eleven attitudes that define the central features of a critical thinker or how a successful critical thinker approaches a problem:

- **Confidence** (belief in oneself)
- **Independent thought** (considering other ideas and concepts before forming an opinion)
- **Fairness** (justly dealing with a situation)
- **Responsibility** and accountability (knowledge that you are accountable for your decisions, actions, and critical thinking)
- **Risk-taking** (leads to advances in care)
- **Discipline** (misses few details, is orderly or systematic when collecting information)
- **Perseverance** (determination to find effective solutions)
- **Creativity** (finding solutions outside the standard routines of care while following standards of practice)
- **Curiosity** (asking "why?" and "what if?")
- **Integrity** (questioning and testing their own knowledge and beliefs)
- **Humility** (admitting limitations in knowledge and skill) (p. 199-205)

Professional standards for critical thinking refer to ethical criteria for nursing judgments, evidence-based criteria used for evaluation, and criteria for professional responsibility. Excellent nursing practice is a reflection of ethical standards. Nurses routinely use evidence-based criteria to assess patients' conditions and determine the efficacy of nursing interventions.

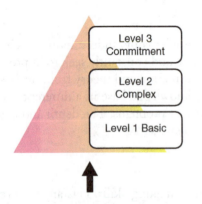

As demonstrated in the diagram, critical thinking is acquired through experience and nursing competency, commitment to learning and developing your foundational knowledge, regular use, and a true understanding of professional standards as well as the mindsets that affect how the nurse approaches a problem.

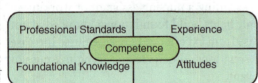

Reflection

Critical thinking is not a simple step-by-step linear process that is learned in a short time; it also involves deep reflection. Reflection involves playing a situation over in your mind so as to carefully and honestly review everything that happened. When we reflect in clinical situations, we often discover new details, improve the accuracy of diagnostic conclusions, and find deeper meaning that corrects and clarifies our own actions, responses, and behaviors. We ask ourselves: How did I act? What could I have done differently? What should I do next time when faced with a similar situation? A critical thinker considers what is important in each clinical situation, reflects on past experiences, looks for new knowledge and explores alternatives, considers ethical principles, and makes informed decisions about the care of patients.

If you would like to learn more about reflective nursing practice, see Jacobs (2016).

Levels of Critical Thinking for Nursing

Basic

In Level 1 critical thinking, a learner trusts that experts have the right answers for every problem. Thinking is concrete and based on a set of rules or principles. A basic critical thinker learns to accept the diverse opinions and values of experts (e.g., instructors, staff nurses, preceptors). Students who enter nursing school are generally at the basic critical thinking level and work to develop, over time, a bridge to Level 2. Nursing faculty look for this mental growth and measure this ability through coursework and clinical assignments. However, inexperience, weak competencies, and inflexible attitudes can restrict a person's ability to move to the next level of critical thinking and is often reflected not only in program course grading but also in the student's ability to understand increasingly complex nursing practice.

Complex

Level 2 critical thinkers begin to separate themselves from their dependence on experts. By the time you are ready to graduate from nursing school, the graduate nurse should safely be operating at this level of critical thought. Nurses operating on the second level are able to analyze the clinical situation and examine choices more independently. In complex critical thinking, each solution has benefits and risks that are weighed before making a final decision because there are options. Thinking becomes more creative and innovative, and the complex critical thinker is willing to consider different options from routine procedures when complex situations develop. Here, the nurse learns to gather additional information and take a variety of different approaches for the same therapy.

Commitment

At the highest level of critical thinking, Level 3, nurses anticipate when to make choices without assistance from others and accept accountability for decisions made. A nurse will do more than just consider the complex alternatives that a problem poses and work to choose actions or beliefs that are based on the available alternatives. Because they take accountability for the decision, nurses at this level consider the results of the decision and determine whether it was appropriate. This is the level of the fully competent RN, practicing fully within their scope and using lifelong learning and evidence-based practice to accurately deliver care. At this level, critical thinking becomes a way of thinking about a situation that always asks, "Why?" "What am I missing?" "What do I really know about this patient's situation?" and "What are my options?" The use of evidence-based knowledge, or knowledge based on research or clinical expertise, makes you an informed Level 3 critical thinker. Critical thinking requires cognitive skills and the habit of asking questions, staying well informed, being honest in facing personal biases, and always being willing to reconsider and think clearly about issues. Nurses who apply critical thinking in their work focus on options for solving problems and making decisions rather than rapidly and carelessly forming quick, simple solutions. Critical thinking is more than just problem-solving. It is a continuous attempt to improve how to apply yourself when faced with problems in patient care and why the RN is licensed and trained in these skills.

Developing Critical Thinking Skills

Developing critical thinking in nursing school specifically involves the use of several educational tools designed to improve your ability to demonstrate and increase critical thinking. The following are examples of these assignments and a brief description of their use in nursing practice.

Critical Thinking Educational Tools	
Reflective Journaling	Allows the nurse to define, explore, and synthesize experiences by returning to an event or series of events through thoughtful reflection
Clinical Case Pre- and Post-Conference	By meeting with colleagues, faculty, as well as other disciplines to discuss a clinical case, nurses gain insight, learn to work as a team, examine work experience, and validate decisions
Concept Mapping	Allows the nurse to create visual representations of relationships between patient problems, nursing diagnoses, interventions

Helpful Reflection Questions for Clinical Situations
Which experience, situation, or information in your clinical experience is confusing, difficult, or interesting?
What is the meaning of the experience?
What feelings did you have?
What feelings did your patient or family have?
What influenced the experience?
Do the feelings, guesses, or questions remind you of any experiences from the past or something that you think is a desirable future experience?
How does it relate?
What are the connections between what is being described and what you have learned about nursing science and theory?

Concept Mapping

In nursing school, you will learn extensively how to create a concept map, not only as a demonstration of your ability to critically think through the nursing process and plan of care for assigned patients but also as a mechanism to show relationships and influences in leadership, community health, health care administration, and ethics. Concept mapping is a nonlinear picture of a patient or situation to be used for comprehensive care planning or analysis.

> In the clinical setting, the primary purpose of concept mapping is to better synthesize relevant data about a patient, including assessment data, nursing diagnoses, health needs, nursing interventions, and evaluation measures.

> Mapping organizes or connects information in a unique way so the diverse information that you have about a patient begins to form meaningful patterns and concepts.

Chapter 4 The Art and Science of Nursing

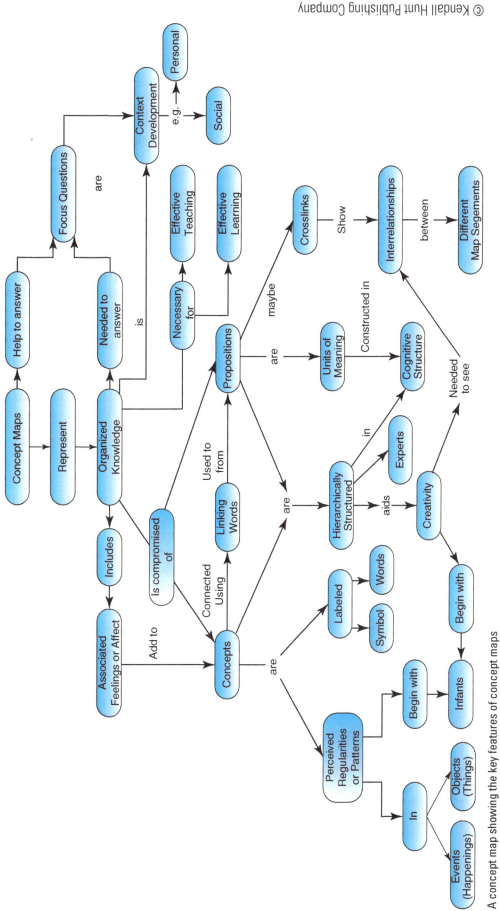

A concept map showing the key features of concept maps

Decision-Making

Decision-making is a product of critical thinking that focuses on problem resolution. Decision-making is different from problem-solving in that solving a problem denotes evaluating a situation over time, identifying possible solutions, and trying a solution to make sure that it is effective. It becomes necessary to try different options if a problem recurs.

In decision-making, there are generally criteria that are used when determining the correct action. These criteria help to make a thorough and thoughtful decision. The criteria may be personal; based on an organizational policy; or, in the case of nursing, a professional standard. The person has to weigh each option against these criteria, test possible options, consider the consequences, and make a final decision. Decision-making involves moving back and forth when considering all criteria. It leads to informed conclusions that are supported by evidence and reason.

Diagnostic Reasoning

Diagnostic reasoning is the analytical process for determining a patient's health problems. Accurate recognition of a patient's problems is necessary before a nurse decides on solutions and implements actions. It requires the RN to assign meaning to the behaviors and physical signs and symptoms presented by a patient. An expert nurse, operating at the highest level of critical thought, sees the context of a patient situation, observes patterns and themes, and makes decisions quickly. Part of diagnostic reasoning is clinical inference, the process of drawing conclusions from related pieces of evidence and previous experience with the evidence. When making an inference, you form patterns of information from data before making a diagnosis. When uncertain of a diagnosis, continue data collection. You have to critically analyze changing clinical situations until you are able to determine a patient's unique situation. Clinical decision-making makes a decision that identifies the problem, reducing the severity of the problem or resolving the problem completely.

Skilled clinical decision-making occurs through in-depth knowledge of a patient's patterns of responses within a clinical situation and knowing the patient as a person. It has two components: a nurse's understanding of a specific patient and his or her subsequent selection of interventions.

Nurses use both the art and the science of nursing when solving clinical problems. The concepts are inseparable. Despite working on a physiological concern, recall that nurses are equally invested in the mind and spirit, a holistic view. Although nurses are trained to improve physical health, it is critical to understand that skilled clinical decision-making involves a balance, requires prioritization of needs, and considers all possible outcomes before taking action.

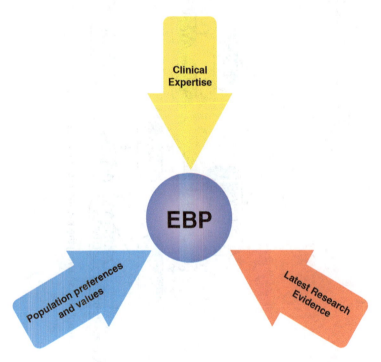

Evidence-based Practice (EBP)

Although it is imperative that nurses synthesize the art and science of nursing into fluid patient care, nurses must ensure that what we do, the actual clinical interventions we provide to patients and families, is based on evidence that our care reflects the most current, highly effective, and safe practice. This can be accomplished only through rigorous, scientific inquiry. If nurses do not abide by the most rigorous research methods and standards, how can we, as a profession, be confident that nursing science is reliable? In addition, in order to shape practice, we must also base practice changes on data that is replicated and applicable across all populations and geographic locations and settings. Within nursing research, this includes data from nursing interventions. Within medical research, this may include data from studies regarding medications or procedures. Within the social sciences, these data include research on communication techniques, interactions, and therapies.

EBPFormally introduced to health care in medicine in 1992, evidence-based practice has steadily been significantly impacting patient care practice in many fields, including nursing. The American Nurses Association (2020) has predicted that evidence-based research findings are now the basis for approximately 90% of current nursing practice. But what is it exactly? By definition, according to Newhouse, Dearholt, Poe, Pugh, and White (2005), evidence-based practice is

> a problem-solving approach to clinical decision-making within a health care organization. It integrates the best available scientific evidence with the best available experiential (patient and practitioner) evidence. EBP considers internal and external influences on practice and encourages critical thinking in the judicious application of such evidence to the care of individual patients, a patient population, or a system (p. 36).

Comprised of four main components, evidence-based practice focuses on the following criteria:

The validity of the research, the reliability of the research, the relevance, and the ultimate outcome of the study.

If the research being reviewed does not meet these criteria, then using it to change a nursing practice would be ineffective. Evaluating each practice must always be done in a way that is mindful of the current practice's proven track record of efficiency, effectiveness, and beneficial or intended positive outcome. However, failing to review nursing practices to ensure that we are using the most current and efficacious methods would consequentially lead to negative or poor patient outcomes. To further explore the concepts involved in evidence-based research, see: http://nursingplanet.com/Nursing_Research/.

Formulating an Evidence-based Clinical Question Using PICO/T

Despite the form of research, the acronym PICO/T is commonly used in nursing *to shape or focus clinical questions* using an evidence-based framework that is based on the literature review you conduct before attempting to ask the question. After all, how can you ask a question if you first haven't looked to see what has already been studied in the nursing literature? **NOTE:** The goal is to influence nursing practice by making sure we are doing the latest and most effective interventions or treatments.

	PICO/T: Designing a Strong Research Question	
P	Patient Population	Whom is the study centered on?
I	Intervention/treatment	What is the intervention or treatment that you are interesting in learning about?
C	Comparison	Is there an alternative to the intervention that you can compare in your study?
O	Outcome/s	What is/are the expected clinical outcome/s?
T	Time* Not always required	What is the period of time it might take to get the outcome?

In clinical practice, health care providers have two basic types of questions known as Background and Foreground questions. This is an important concept for student nurses because everything you are about to learn will seem new to you, and yet there is a difference between the kind of questions and material found in your textbooks and information that is specific to nursing care. Background questions are generally answered in textbooks; they are the kinds of questions that establish general knowledge. Background questions become the foundation on which you may pose a clinical or Foreground question. For example, Background questions usually begin with "when" or "what," whereas Foreground questions generally begin with "how." Let's use an example. If we are talking about low blood sugar in patients (we call this hypoglycemia), we might ask *What* are the signs and symptoms of someone who has hypoglycemia. When we provide the answer to this question, you begin to form the foundation of your understanding of the concept; it provides you with a general understanding. But let us now shift to an example of a Foreground question, a question that we would put into the PICO/T format because we are focusing on a clinical issue *related to* the information we learned on hypoglycemia. In Type II diabetic patients over 40 years old, do weekly dietary education sessions compared with monthly dietary education sessions lower the incidence of hypoglycemia, over a 6-month period? Now we have a Foreground question because, when we answer the question, it helps us provide evidence on which we can base a clinical practice decision. In our example, if we conducted the study carefully, might we be able to determine whether one intervention was better than the other in improving a patient outcome?

Let's take our Foreground question and apply the PICO/T system to see if we have a strong research question: In Type II diabetic patients over 40 years old (P), do weekly dietary education sessions (I) compared with monthly dietary education sessions (C) lower the incidence of hypoglycemia (O) over a 6-month period (T)?

To help you understand how this is done, review the following templates from Melnyk and Fineout-Overholt (2011). These templates have helped clinicians all over the world ensure they formulate their Foreground questions appropriately.

> When creating a research question for an **INTERVENTION**, try the following question template:
>
> In _____(P), how does _____ (I) compared with _____ (C) affect _____(O) within _____(T)?
>
> When creating a research question that involves a **PREDICTION OR PROGNOSIS**, try the following question template:
>
> In _____ (P), how does _____ (I) compared with _____ (C) influence/predict _____(O) over _____(T)?
>
> When creating a research question involving a **DIAGNOSIS OR DIAGNOSTIC TEST**, try the following question template:
>
> In _____ (P), are/is _____ (I) compared with _____(C) more accurate in diagnosing _____(O)?
>
> When creating a research question involving an **ETIOLOGY**, try the following question template:
>
> Are _____ (P), who have _____ (I) compared with those without _____ (C) at _____ risk for/of _____(O) over _____(T)?
>
> When creating a research question involving the **MEANING** of a concept, try the following question template:
>
> How do _____(P) with _____ (I) perceive _____ (O) during _____(T)?
>
> Source: Melnyk, B. M., & Fineout-Overholt, E. (2011). *Evidence-based practice in nursing and healthcare: A guide to best practice* (2nd ed.). Philadelphia, PA: Lippincott Williams & Wilkins.

Evidence-based Practice Models

It is a bit easier to conceive of what a concept involves when all of its components are placed in a model. One of the best models available comes from Johns Hopkins. Here, we see yet another representation of how evidenced-based practice is organized with the material requiring a critical review (either research or other nonresearch clinical processes) at the center; influenced by practice, education, and research; and influenced by both external and internal factors. Internal factors include culture, the environment, the available equipment and supplies, the number of staff available, and standards of care; whereas external factors include regulatory agencies such as accreditation and legislative bodies, industry regulations, and standards and quality measures.

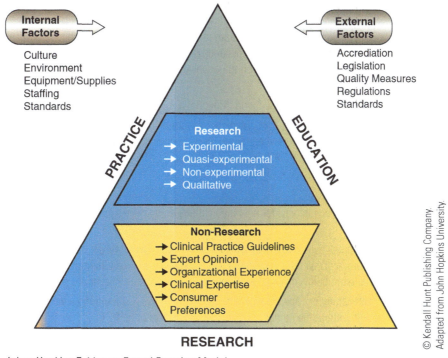

Johns Hopkins Evidence-Based Practice Model

Levels of Evidence

The preceding graphic helps illustrate the hierarchy involving the rigor of research in evidence-based nursing practice. By simply looking at the levels, which level would be most significant? Isn't the top of the pyramid generally seen as the highest point? Naturally, then, it follows that a graphic, including a pyramid, correlates the most significant level of evidence and highest level of quality (or Level I), followed logically by Level II, Level III, Level IV, and, finally, Level V. According to the Evidence Based Practice Toolkit from Winona State University (2020), "Levels of evidence (sometimes called hierarchy of evidence) are assigned to studies based on the methodological quality of their design, validity, and applicability to patient care. These decisions gives the 'grade (or strength) of recommendation' (Levels of Evidence, Para, 1). https://libguides.winona.edu/c.php?g=11614&p=61584

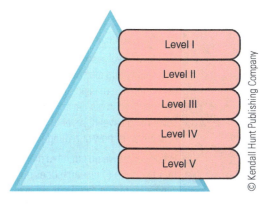

Consider a new policy that your hospital has written on how to care for people with a contagious virus. Would you feel more comfortable knowing that the policy was based on research that was considered Level I and Level II evidence, or would you feel comfortable implementing the policy knowing that the evidence used to develop the policy was solely from Level V? The stronger the evidence, the more efficacious the outcome. Basically, evidence is ranked or stacked from least quality to best quality. Each level of evidence is therefore comprised of different forms of research or support. Sometimes, it isn't research but rather a pattern of interventions that have successfully worked serially over time; sometimes "nonresearch" support involving expert opinion or reports from expert committees, or specific qualitative themes. Each level of evidence is described in the following table based on Dang and Dearholt (2017).

Level	Description
Level I	This level is the highest, most rigorous, highest quality level and includes evidence from random control trials (called RCTs) or a meta-analysis of an RCT (using statistics and combining data from multiple studies to look for a common effect). An RCT is a clinical study in which participants are randomly (by chance) assigned to one of several possible interventions. There are usually hundreds to thousands of participants. This is what researchers call "true research" because there is a specific research question that involves a causal relationship. By manipulating the variables, researchers derive a specific outcome. An example of an RCT in nursing can be found through the following citation: Austin, A. L., Spalding, C. N., Landa, K. N., Myer, B. R., Cure, D., Smith, J. E., Platt, G., & King, H. C. (2020). A randomized control trial of cardiopulmonary feedback devices and their impact on infant chest compression quality. *Pediatric Emergency Care, 36*(2), e79–e84 doi: 10.1097/PEC.0000000000001312 https://journals.lww.com/pec-online/Abstract/2020/02000/A_Randomized_Control_Trial_of_Cardiopulmonary.21.aspx You may have seen RCT commercials for new medications or cancer treatment? Here is a video example https://youtu.be/fkOCYov1p-o
Level II	This level involves studies called quasi-experimental. This level is also rated as having good quality or reasonably consistent results and can involve systematic reviews of quasi-experimental studies as well as other RCTs or meta-analysis. (See table below on difference between systematic and literature reviews). A quasi-experimental study is a special kind of study that involves manipulating a variable (a factor that can be changed or adapted) without the random assignment that is part of an RCT. An example of a quasi-experimental research design used in a nursing study can be found through the following citation: Bas-Sarmiento, P., Fernβndez-Gutiérrez, M., Baena-Baños, M., & Romero-Sβnchez, J.M. (2017). Efficacy of empathy training in nursing students: A quasi-experimental study. *Nurse Education Today, 59*, 59–65. doi:10.1016/j.nedt.2017.08.012 https://pubmed.ncbi.nlm.nih.gov/28945994/ Here is a quick video example to help explain the difference between a quasi-experimental study and a true experiment like an RCT in Level I: https://youtu.be/vm-7k6unuLo
Level III	This level involves nonexperimental studies and systematic reviews of nonexperimental studies. It is considered low quality and may have inconsistent results. A nonexperimental study is a group of studies that, by definition, do not include manipulation of an independent variable, as seen in our Level II studies, and also lacks randomization, as seen in our Level I studies. This can be an either or both scenario. The biggest distinction is that unlike Level I and Level II, Level III evidence does not involve a causation. Level III studies compare and describe, but a conclusion of how one thing leads to another is not the purpose of this level of research evidence. Even though we do not have manipulation of variables, as we do in true experimental research, it does not mean that this form of research does not have value. Sometimes, the topics we want to study include variables that cannot be manipulated either because of an ethical concern (we cannot ethically withhold specific care from one group over another) or because they simply cannot technically be accomplished (such as attempting to manipulate variables such as birth weight, body temperature, or ethnicity).

	Basically, at this level we see research that allows researchers to observe a phenomenon naturally without introducing any variables or controlling the setting. Often, the purpose of nonexperimental research designs allows exploration and description of phenomena, allows nursing to develop theories and identify problems, and also allows us to determine what others in similar situations might be doing with regard to a topic, condition, or issue. It is commonly the precursor to experimental research as well. Here is a citation involving a nonexperimental research design. Note that this study involves a comparative approach, which is one form of nonexperimental research: Joseph, J. M. (2015). *A correlational study between the hospital patient safety culture and computer self-efficacy among nurses in a hospital.* A Dissertation. Retrieved from https://rucore.libraries.rutgers.edu/rutgers-lib/48234/PDF/1/play/ Here is a quick video example of qualitative nonexperimental research: https://youtu.be/10nMNh3RMp0
Level IV	Level IV involves expert opinions based on scientific evidence, clinical practice guidelines (recommendation statements by experts usually in the form of a systematic review of the literature on a topic with the sole purpose of improving or optimizing patient care), or consensus panels (statement by a group of experts agreeing on evidence-based knowledge and practice). Level IV can contain a range of quality, from high quality to low quality, depending on the material. Many examples of actual clinical practice guidelines can be found using the National Center for Complementary and Integrative health (NIH) Clinical Practice database using the following link: https://www.nccih.nih.gov/health/providers/clinicalpractice An example of a consensus panel: The American Geriatrics Society and American Association for Geriatric Psychiatry Expert Panel on Quality Mental Health Care in Nursing Homes developed the following consensus statement on Improving the quality of mental health care in U.S. nursing homes: https://onlinelibrary.wiley.com/doi/abs/10.1046/j.1532-5415.2003.51415.x Here is a video that describes what a clinical practice guideline is and how they are used: https://youtu.be/MmjVo0wYzsQ
Level V	The fifth level of evidence involves literature reviews, quality improvement projects for clinical agencies, evaluations of programs and financial documents, case reports, as well as opinions of experts based on experimental evidence. Level V can also contain a range of quality, from high quality to low quality, depending on the material. Note: ** the comparison table below of the difference between a systematic review and a literature review. They are not the same!** Literature reviews are a survey of scholarly books, articles, theses, dissertations, and so on to reveal existing knowledge on a given topic or focused question. Literature reviews allow nurses to easily identify the gaps in research or the areas where there is little to no evidence available. For more on Nursing Literature Review (2020) see: https://nsufl.libguides.com/c.php?g=112208&p=3381901 See the following example of a nursing literature review: Labrague, L. J., McEnroe-Petitte, D. M., Gloe, D., Thomas, L., Papathanasiou, I. V., & Tsaras, K. (2017). A literature review on stress and coping strategies in nursing students. *Journal of Mental Health, 26*(5), 471–480. https://www.tandfonline.com/doi/abs/10.1080/09638237.2016.1244721 Quality improvement projects have been around for decades and have gone by different acronyms, depending on the era. Basically, it is a formal systematic approach to improving performance in an organization. Quality improvement projects on nursing floors in hospitals have included reduction of patient falls or improving nursing student experiences in clinical. See the following example of a quality improvement project: Levett-Jones, T., Fahy, K., Parsons, K., & Mitchell, A. (2006). Enhancing nursing students' clinical placement experiences: A quality improvement project. *Contemporary Nurse, 23*(1), 58–71. https://www.tandfonline.com/doi/abs/10.5172/conu.2006.23.1.58

	Systematic Review	Literature Review
Definition	• High-level overview of primary research on a focused question that identifies, selects, synthesizes, and appraises all high-quality research evidence relevant to that question.	• Qualitatively summarizes evidence on a topic using informal or subjective methods to collect and interpret studies.
Goals	• Answer a focused clinical question • Eliminate bias	• Provide summary or overview of topic
Question	• Clearly defined and answerable clinical question • Recommend using PICO as a guide	• Can be a general topic or a specific question
Components	• Prespecified eligibility criteria • Systematic search strategy • Assessment of the validity of findings • Interpretation and presentation of results • Reference list	• Introduction • Methods • Discussion • Conclusion • Reference list
Number of Authors	• Three or more	• One or more
Timeline	• Months to years • Average eighteen months	• Weeks to months
Requirements	• Thorough knowledge of topic • Perform searches of all relevant databases • Statistical analysis resources (for meta-analysis)	• Understanding of topic • Perform searches of one or more databases
Value	• Connects practicing clinicians to high-quality evidence • Supports evidence-based practice	• Provides summary of literature on a topic

Source: Adapted from Norris Medical Library (2020).

There are a number of research search engines for nursing. The most helpful nursing research search engine involves TRIP (Turning Evidence Into Practice). Throughout nursing school and nursing practice, you will need to become well acquainted with search engines and levels of evidence to support your nursing practice. See the following guide on databases used for specific forms of research such as systematic reviews, RCTs, case reports and expert opinions: https://libguides.daemen.edu/EBP/search/levels-of-evidence

As a nursing student, you will have an entire course on nursing research so that you will become adept at scholarly critical appraisal and conducting research.

See the following handout from Ohio State University taken from Dearholt and Dang (2012).

What Makes a Good Research Study?

First, nurses look for gaps in the literature…this means we look for areas that have little to no research conducted on the issue or topic. For example, although we might have a significant amount of research on the use of massage in adult and pediatric patient care, perhaps we find no body of research available on how massage impacts cultures in which touch and personal space are considered private or intimate. Second, nurses work to ensure that the research question they develop captures the content area missing in the expanse of available data. When we formulate a research question, we want to make sure that the question is important, that it is something that can be answered using a chosen research method, and that it is not only ethical to conduct but also feasible. "Feasible" refers to something that is easily done or probable. So how do we decide what kind of research method to use when we develop a great question? The answer lies in learning about the different forms of research discussed next. Once you understand the different kinds of research and what we use them for in nursing, you will unlock tremendous potential in your nursing career.

Forms of Research

There are two main forms of research: Quantitative and Qualitative Research. Although there are occasions when nurses find that the outcome would better be served by a bit of both, something we call Mixed Method, for this basic introduction to nursing research we will leave it simple. Let's take a look at the two main forms of research side by side.

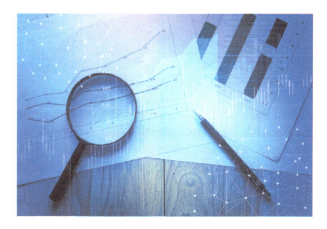 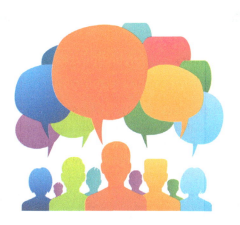

Quantitative	Qualitative
Involves deductive reasoning	Involves inductive reasoning
Expressed in numbers	Expressed in words
Objective	Subjective
Comprehensive	Specific
Large sample size	Smaller sample size
Systematic	Systematic

Quantitative

There are three types of quantitative research:

- **correlational research** https://www.questionpro.com/blog/correlational-research/
- **quasi-experimental research** https://conjointly.com/kb/quasi-experimental-design/
- **descriptive research** http://members.aect.org/edtech/ed1/41/41-01.html

Quantitative research contains four basic components: a hypothesis; a study group where all share common features; a variable or variables, which could be anything we want to introduce, such as a nursing intervention, a medication, or a product; and, finally, an outcome, that is, what are we expecting to happen? A hypothesis should always explain what you expect to happen, it's your prediction; it should be clear, specific, and understandable; it should be something that can be tested and measured; and it should contain independent and dependent variables.

Qualitative

Qualitative research is used to generate new knowledge or to support existing knowledge and is focused on a participant's thoughts, feelings, and experiences. The unique feature of qualitative research is that it may not have an outcome because researchers are using this form to simply gain further insight into a situation or concept. As in quantitative research, there are also basic components but they are different. These components include a hypothesis or theory, an observation that occurs through an experience, a practice-based intervention/s, and strategies for implementation, and is approached either using a traditional, more formal method or can be done casually. Qualitative research generally also includes relevant background or circumstances that have influenced the participant and allows for unique variation as well as the potential of adverse reactions. There are five types of qualitative research. Visit the following URLs to learn more about how and why the method is used.

Phenomenology https://ebn.bmj.com/content/21/4/96

Historical Research https://libguides.usc.edu/humanitiesresearch/historical

Symbolic Interactionism https://methods.sagepub.com/reference/the-sage-encyclopedia-of-communication-research-methods/i14544.xml

Grounded Theory https://ebn.bmj.com/content/19/2/34

Ethnography https://ebn.bmj.com/content/20/4/98

The researcher selects the type of research method on the basis of the study envisioned. For instance, if you were interested in learning about the experience that the junior nursing students had while on a study abroad mission trip, a survey might work, but that would indicate that you had a range of possible answers for how they experienced the trip. What if you thought they all had positive feelings about their travels, and you did not account for this in your survey answer choices? Your result would be a biased study, which reflects only what you anticipated as responses. It might make more sense to use a phenomenological approach, meaning you are generally interested in learning what the trip meant to each person. By understanding how each of your peers experienced the trip, you could use these data to better inform the experience of your peers next year.

Nursing is full of acronyms to help us remember concepts. Like PICO/T, an acronym used to help you remember how to create a proper research question, we like to use the acronym DIDACTIC to help us remember *what to do when conducting an actual study.*

 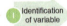   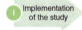 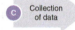

© Kendall Hunt Publishing Company

D stands for developing the hypothesis
I stands for identification of the common variables
D stands for the research design
A stands for acquiring the data that is pertinent to your study
C stands for communication. We must always remember to communicate the goals of the study with every member of the health care team
T stands for talking. We must equally ensure that we are talking with the people who have agreed to be in the study so that we know they are fully informed of the potential risks, benefits, and goals of the study to their person. These people are called "research participants."
I stands for implementation of the study. Once we have obtained each participant's signed consent to participate in the study, we begin!
C is the final letter in the mnemonic and stands for collection. Collect your data and evaluate it using the correct method so that you can write the outcome or conclusion of your study and share it with your peers.

Research Terminology

Although the idea of research seems daunting, we must, as with learning medical terminology, work to understand what we are reading. What is the special language used in research? Once we learn the key concepts and words, research becomes part of our everyday clinical practice. Let's take a moment to review and contextualize some of the key research terms. Additional glossary definitions of terminology and concepts common to nursing, research, and health care can be found through the Agency for Healthcare Research and Quality (AHRQ) website, glossary: https://psnet.ahrq.gov/glossary

Summary

In this chapter, the role of the professional nurse is twofold: artful care and scientific competency. Providing exceptional care artfully with value, dignity, and respect blended with a solid, scientific foundation leads nurses to competence, quality, and excellence in care, research, and future practice. This chapter exposed the learner to the essential components of critical thinking in nursing practice. Learners discovered the value of reflection and understood the components of gaining high-level critical thinking ability for use across all nursing settings. The use of reflection journaling, concept maps, and the role of pre- and post-conference in the clinical setting brought to the fore the need for students in nursing programs to use experience, knowledge, values, and attitudes as well as opportunity, to grow to their full potential. Evidence-based practice and the forms of research were explored as being central to nursing science and the future of health care. As such, learners were also introduced to the PICOT format in the development of clinical research questions and the multiple forms of research that can be used to further nursing science.

References

Brenan, M. (2018). *Nurses again outpace other professions for honesty, ethics.* Retrieved from https://news.gallup.com/poll/245597/nurses-again-outpace-professions-honesty-eth

Curtis, K. (2015). Compassion is an essential component of good nursing care and can be conveyed through the smallest actions. *Evidence-Based Nursing, 18*(95), 2790–2799.

Dang, D., & Dearholt, S. (2017). *Johns Hopkins nursing evidence-based practice: Model and guidelines* (3rd ed.). Indianapolis, IN: Sigma Theta Tau International. Retrieved from www.hopkinsmedicine.org/evidence-based-practice/ijhn_2017_ebp.html

Dearholt, S. L., & Dang, D. (2012). *Johns Hopkins nursing evidence-based practice: Models and guidelines* (2nd ed.). Indianapolis, IN: Sigma Theta Tau International. Retrieved from https://libguides.ohsu.edu/ld.php?content_id=16277844

Denzin, N. K., & Lincoln, Y. S. (2011). *The SAGE handbook of qualitative research* (4th ed.). Thousand Oaks, CA: SAGE.

Donahue, M. P. (1996). *Nursing: The finest art: An illustrated history.* St Louis, MO: C.V. Mosby.

Echevarria, I. M., & Walker, S. (2014). To make your case, start with a PICOT question. *Nursing, 44*(2), 18–19. doi:10.1097/01.NURSE.0000442594.00242.f9

Glasofer, A., & Townsend, A. B. (2020a). Determining the level of evidence: Nonexperimental research designs. *Nursing Critical Care, 15*(1), 24–27.

Glasofer, A., & Townsend, A. B. (2020b). Determining the level of evidence. *Nursing Critical Care, 15*(2), 22–26. doi:10.1097/01.CCN.0000654792.71629.00

Grove, S. K., & Burns, N. (2008). *The practice of nursing research: Appraisal, synthesis, and generation of evidence* (6th ed.). St. Louis, MO: Elsevier Saunders.

Hack, L., & Gwyer, J. (2013). *Evidence into practice: Integrating judgment, values, and research.* Philadelphia, PA: F.A. Davis.

Jacobs, S. (2016). Reflective learning, reflective practice. *Nursing, 46*(5), 62–64. doi:10.1097/01.NURSE.0000482278.79660.f2; Retrieved from https://journals.lww.com/nursing/FullText/2016/05000/Reflective_learning,_reflective_practice.18.aspx

Kataoka-Yahiro, M., & Saylor, C. (1994). A critical thinking model for nursing judgement. *Journal of Nursing Education, 33*(8), 351.

Keltner, D. (2009). *Born to be good: The science of a meaningful life.* New York, NY: W.W. Norton.

Leininger, M. M. (1991). *Culture care diversity and universality: A theory of nursing.* New York, NY: National League of Nursing Press.

McCance, T. V., McKenna, H. P., & Boore, J. R. P. (1999). Caring: Theoretical perspectives of relevance to nursing. *Journal of Advanced Nursing, 30*(6), 1388–1396.

Melnyk, B. M., Fineout-Overholt, E., Gallagher-Ford, L., & Kaplan, L. (2012). The state of evidence-based practice in US nurses: Critical implications for nurse leaders and educators. *Journal of Nursing Administration, 42*(9), 410–417.

Melnyk, B. M., & Fineout-Overholt, E. (2011). *Evidence-based practice in nursing and healthcare: A guide to best practice* (2nd ed.). Philadelphia, PA: Lippincott Williams & Wilkins.

Melnyk, B. M., & Fineout-Overholt, E. (2019). *Evidence-based practice in nursing and healthcare: A guide to best practice* (4th ed.). Philadelphia, PA: Wolters Kluwer.

Melnyk, B. M., Fineout-Overholt, E., Stillwell, S. B., & Williamson, K. M. (2010). Evidence-based practice: Step by step: The seven steps of evidence-based practice. *American Journal of Nursing, 110*(1), 51–53.

Munhall, P. L. (2010). *Nursing research: A qualitative perspective* (5th ed.). Sudbury, MA: Jones & Bartlett Learning.

Newhouse, R., Dearholt, S., Poe, S., Pugh, L., & White, K. M. (2005). Evidence-based practice: A practical approach to implementation. *Journal of Nursing Administration, 35*(1), 35–40.

NursingPlanet.com. (n.d.). *Qualitative research in nursing.* Retrieved from https://nursingplanet.com/research/qualitative_research.html

Pangarakis, S., & Graner, T. (2010). Engage nurses in EBP with the nursing clinical question process. *Nursing Management, 41*(6), 15–17.

Parse, R. R. (1989). Essentials for practicing the art of nursing. *Nursing Science Quarterly, 2*(3), 111.

Polit, D. F., & Beck, C. T. (2011). *Nursing research: Generating and assessing evidence for nursing practice* (9th ed.). Philadelphia, PA: Lippincott Williams & Wilkins.

Potter, P. A., Griffin-Perry, A., Stockert, P., & Hall, A. (2013). Critical thinking in nursing practice. In *Fundamentals of nursing e-book* (8th ed.). Philadelphia, PA: Elsevier Health Sciences.

Schantz, M. L. (2007). Compassion: A concept analysis. *Nursing Forum, 42,* 48–55. doi:10.1111/j.1744-6198.2007.00067.x

Schoenhofer, S. O. (2002). Choosing personhood: Intentionality and the theory of nursing as caring. *Holistic Nursing Practice, 16*(4), 36–40.

Stillwell, S. B., Fineout-Overholt, E., Melnyk, B. M., & Williamson, K. M. (2010). Evidence-based practice, step by step: Asking the clinical question: A key step in evidence-based practice. *American Journal of Nursing, 110*(3), 58–61.

Torres, G. (1990). The place of concepts and theories within nursing. In J. B. George (Ed.). *Nursing theories: The base for professional nursing practice* (3rd ed.). Norwalk, CT: Appleton & Lange.

Venes, D. (2020). *Taber's cyclopedic medical dictionary* (23rd ed.). Philadelphia, PA: F. A. Davis.

Watson, J. (2008). *Nursing: The philosophy and science of caring* (Rev. ed.). Boulder: University Press of Colorado.

Wolcott, H. F. (2008). *Writing up qualitative research* (3rd ed.). Newbury Park, CA: SAGE.

Chapter 5

Foundations in Nursing Theory

Chapter Objectives:

- Understand why theory is an important component of all professions.
- Discuss the difference between the levels of theory and the rationale for each.
- Identify important nursing theorists and how they shaped nursing.
- Identify the link between nursing theory, research, and practice.

Within any discipline, science forms at the intersection of inquiry (research) and knowledge (theory) (Saleh, 2018). In nursing, research subsequently guides nursing practice by building knowledge through the creation of theory and empirical theory testing. In a reciprocal fashion, we also know that theory provides a framework of perspective that guides research. Together, these concepts influence how we provide care to patients both through evidence and through knowledge. Although it seems that nurses rarely use the term 'theory' in practice, there remains a triangular relationship between the three cornerstones (research, theory, and practice) within our discipline.

As a basic introduction to nursing theory, we will discuss a general overview of each kind of theory so as to form a foundation of understanding. According to Petiprin (2016), nursing theory is defined as "a belief, policy, or procedure proposed or followed as the basis of action. Nursing theory is an organized framework of concepts and purposes designed to guide the practice of nursing" (Nursing Theory Definition, para 1). Think back to the lives of the nurses in Chapter 2. As nursing evolved, many of these nurses took action to advance nursing because they found it difficult to define how and why nursing care was conducted in a specific way. They fought for formalized training and more defined rigorous education. They looked at the evidence and what was improving outcomes. Slowly, nurses found it essential to write down their beliefs, working to explain and describe nursing care. These concepts were developed into theories and subsequently began guiding nursing practice. Recall Florence Nightingale's keen observation ability and the extreme thought she put into determining the best care for patients during the Crimean War. She stated in *Notes on Nursing* that nursing theory would guide our profession in defining the context of nursing and nursing care (Nightingale, 1859/1992). Today, we have many nursing theories that were designed to explain different aspects of patient care, such as self-care, adaptation, and culture care diversity. Nursing theories conceptualize all aspects of nursing, describing, explaining, and even predicting nursing practice. Theory provides nurses with an ontology or way to view the world. Think about putting on clear lens glasses and looking around. The world seems clear and bright. Now put on a pair of glasses that are tinted blue. How does the world appear? The world is the same, and yet our view is a bit different. Theory gives us the means to care for patients using different lenses and affords us unlimited practice potential.

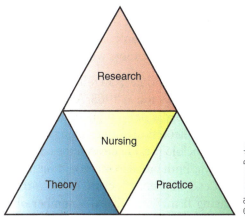

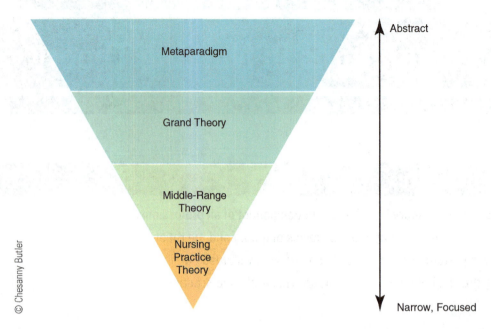

There are many different theories that are created for different reasons, and nursing has grouped them into three distinct levels. Nursing theories are divided into: Grand Theory, Middle-Range Theory, and Nursing Practice Theory. Let's take a moment to begin developing in our minds a visual that will exemplify how to think of the relationship and effect of nursing theory. Picture a growing tree from root to leaves. At the most abstract, and before we can form grand theory, we first understand how theoretical knowledge begins. Have you ever had an idea that when shared with others gains agreement? A new insight perhaps on the way something works? A metaparadigm represents the global perspective or central concepts of the discipline and forms a very general framework from which a conceptual model can be derived (Eckberg & Hill, 1979). Think of a metaparadigm as the seeds of our tree example. It's the very initial ideas, the beliefs of a developing field or discipline, and the basic agreement about an abstract concept that will develop into grand theory. Within nursing, the metaparadigms of person (the recipient of care), environment (all of the conditions that influence the person), health (degree of wellness) and nursing (actions, characteristics, and attributes of the person giving the care) come together abstractly (Flaskerud & Holloran, 1980, cited in Fawcett, 1994). Grand Theories form the roots of the tree. It is what gives nursing practice definition, its scope and strength, and the conceptual model for all of nursing practice. Naturally, out of intention, grand theories have limits, as they seek to explain nursing in a global context but are so broad and all-encompassing that they do not easily allow for empirical testing. Grand Theory helps direct, explain, and predict, as mentioned previously, and is pertinent to all nursing situations. Grand Theories include the foundational works of Leininger (Theory of Culture Care Diversity and Universality), Newman (Theory of Health as Expanding Consciousness), Orem (Self-Care Deficit), Rogers (Science of Unitary Human Beings) and Parse (Theory of Human Becoming). We will discuss these specific theories later in the chapter.

In continuing with our mental visualization of how theories in nursing fit together, close your eyes now and picture our tree. Recall that the seeds represented the metaparadigm and the roots of the tree formed grand nursing theory. Think now for a moment of the trunk and main branches. Middle-Range Theory is the bridge that connects the roots with the leaf forming branches of our living nursing practice.

The idea of Middle-Range Theory, however, was not the original concept of nursing. It was originally proposed by Robert Merton in 1968. Although you might naturally assume that Dr. Merton was a nurse, he was not. The use of theory is not unique to nursing, and, as nursing is a relatively new science, you may be able to imagine that the theoretical underpinnings of other disciplines have been ongoing for centuries. In this case, Dr. Merton was a sociologist. He created the concept of Middle-Range Theory out of a need to devise a theoretical range that was both broad in scope and yet narrow enough to allow empirical testing. Nursing scholars proposed using this level of theory because of the difficulty in testing grand theory within our own discipline (Jacox, 1974). Having firmly established a number of grand theories by the 1970s, the addition of Middle-Range Theory was timely. This theoretical "bridge" between grand theory and bedside nursing practice led to the creation of over 90 Middle-Range Theories between 1988 and 2017 alone (Liehr & Smith, 2018). As noted by American philosopher Frederick Suppe, "as science matures, the development of knowledge moves from grand theory to the development of Middle-Range Theory, because of the decreasing need for abstraction and the increasing need for empirical or practice-based application" (Suppe, as cited in Schmidt, 2004, p. 9). Middle-Range Theory serves as a framework for nurses in providing appropriate health care interventions. It connects grand theory with practice and allows for theory-based research, given a limited number of variables and application. Middle-Range Theories include the work of Dorothy Johnson (Behavioral Systems Model), Katherine Kolcaba (Theory of Comfort), Nola Pender (Health Promotion Model), Merle Mishel (Theory of Uncertainty in Illness), and Ramona Thieme Mercer (Theory of Maternal Role Attainment), to name a few.

Nursing Practice Theory is our final level of nursing theory and forms the multiple and very specific twigs and secondary branches of our visualized tree. Nursing practice forms the ever-changing leaves of our tree. Always growing in new directions, nursing practice theories have the narrowest of scope and level of abstraction/application because they are developed for use within a specific range of nursing situations. Saleh (2018) posits that theory-guided practice, or what we call "Nursing Practice Theory," is the future of nursing. Theory-guided practice shapes the development and implementation of the plan of care and cannot be discerned from one another (p.18). Nursing Practice Theories are interrelated with concepts from middle and grand theory, making them appropriate in addressing specific nursing situations. Think of our tree again; you cannot have living, growing branches and leaves if these leaves and branches are not connected to both the trunk itself and the subsequent roots. They are interrelated. This allows Nursing Practice Theory to be the framework for interventions and helps us predict outcomes for patients. Because nursing practice theories are so narrow in purpose, they are often also defined by a specific specialty, a patient population or a particular community of interest, at a specific time. An example of a Nursing Practice Theory would include the work of Mercer (Becoming a Mother Theory), Beck (Postpartum Depression Theory), Barker (Tidal Model of Mental Health Recovery) and Scheel (Interactional Nursing). Nursing Practice Theory offers different perspectives for patient assessment and helps nurses interpret and organize data, plan effective nursing interventions, and evaluate outcomes. In addition, nursing theory guides nursing research and helps develop new practice.

Theoretical Foundations of Nursing Practice

Some of our most famous nursing theorists, from Grand through Nursing Practice, have been provided for you in this chapter. Let's take a moment to review each of the following Grand Theorists, noting their unique definition of each of the four nursing metaparadigms at https://nurseslabs.com/wp-content/uploads/2019/06/Nursing-Theorist-Metaparadigm-Examples.jpg

Grand Theorists

Florence Nightingale (Environmental Theory of Nursing)	Dorothea Orem (Self-Care Model)
Virginia Henderson (The Nature of Nursing)	Hildegard Peplau (Interpersonal Relations Model)
Martha Rogers (Unitary Human Beings)	Imogene King (Goal Attainment Theory)
Jean Watson (Philosophy and Science of Caring)	Rosemary Parse (Human Becoming Theory)
Sr. Calista Roy (Adaptation Model)	Dorothy Johnson (Behavioral Systems Model)
Fay Abdella (Topology of 21 Nursing Problems)	

One of the best resources for students, when looking for a quick way to understand the basic tenets of any nursing theory, is to read the content on the website Currentnursing.com. This site provides a detailed list of nursing theorists and general overviews of each theory.

See: http://currentnursing.com/nursing_theory/

Summary

As you are probably starting to piece together, everything done in nursing today is based on theory. According to Saleh (2018), "The primary purpose of theory in the profession of nursing is to improve practice by positive influence on the health and quality of life of patients" (p.18). And yet within nursing, just as we rely on other disciplines to provide specialized expertise to patient care, so too do we find the use of theory from other disciplines. A theory is made strongest when multiple disciplines affirm the theoretical application of it within their own fields. Within nursing, you will therefore also find the use of developmental theory, psychosocial theory, stress and adaptation theories from sociology and psychology, systems theory from business, and other health and wellness models. While you learn skills and gain competency, you should ask yourself which theory is being applied to the nursing practice you may be engaged in with your patient. As you remember from Chapter 2, in the early days of American nursing there was little formal nursing knowledge. As nursing education developed, the need to categorize knowledge led to the development of nursing theory to help nurses evaluate increasingly complex client care. Without knowing it, nurses often use a number of theories in their nursing care every day. Knowing what these theories are helps us build a better care environment for our patients. Once you have a firm grasp of theory, you will be able to use the correct theory that best fits the clinical situation. Nursing theory represents insight through different lenses to view, describe, explain, and provide nursing care. They do not compete with one another; rather, they are in concert with one another. Theory provides your roadmap to how you will choose to practice. You will feel reaffirmed in your reasoning for its selection because theory, research, and practice work together to improve patient care, patient outcomes, and nurse–patient communication. Using theory helps us generate new knowledge, which in turn shapes future practice.

References

Eckberg, D. L., & Hill, L., Jr. (1979). The paradigm concept and sociology: A critical review. *American Sociological Review, 44*, 925–937.

Fawcett, J. (1994). *Analysis and evaluation of conceptual models of nursing.* Philadelphia, PA: F. A. Davis.

Jacox, A. (1974). Theory construction in nursing: An overview. *Nursing Research, 23*(1), 4–13.

Liehr, P., & Smith, M. J. (2018). *Middle range theory for nursing* (4th ed.). New York, NY: Springer.

Meleis, A. I. (1991). *Theoretical nursing: Development and progress.* Philadelphia, PA: J. B. Lippincott.

Merton, R. (1968). *Social theory and social structure.* New York, NY: The Free Press.

Nightingale, F. (1992). *Notes on nursing: What it is and what it is not.* Philadelphia, PA: Lippincott. (Original work published 1859)

Parker, M. E. (2005). Introduction to nursing theory. In *Nursing theories & nursing practice* (2nd ed.). Philadelphia, PA: F. A. Davis.

Petiprin, A. (2016). Nursing theory. Retrieved from https://nursing-theory.org/articles/nursing-theory-definition.php

Saleh, U. S. (2018). Theory guided practice in nursing. *Journal of Nursing Research and Practice, 2*(1), 18. Retrieved from https://www.pulsus.com/scholarly-articles/theory-guided-practice-in-nursing.pdf

Schmidt, N. (2004). Response to the pediatric nurse—A societal need. *Self-Care, Dependent-Care and Nursing, 12*(2), 7–9. Retrieved from https://static1.squarespace.com/static/55f1d474e4b03fe7646a4d5d/t/55f35e71e4b0fb5d95ae37c9/1442012785636/Vol12No2Aug2004.pdf

Wayne, G. (2020). *Nursing theories and theorists.* Retrieved from https://nurseslabs.com/nursing-theories/

Part 2: Nursing Communication

Chapter 6

Patient and Health Team Communication

Chapter Objectives

- Why is communication an important component of patient care?
- What are examples of effective therapeutic communication techniques?
- What are the elements of professional communication?
- Distinguish between good and bad professional nursing communication.
- Describe the levels of communication and zones of personal space.
- Describe the components of the communication process.
- Provide examples of the forms of communication. Which communication techniques are required for clients who require alternate communication formats?

Communication and Nursing Practice

Communication. As we begin to explore this topic, you may be wondering how or why communication is a component of a nursing text. After all, haven't we all been communicating in one way or another since birth? We have learned already how to read and write, we have taken English classes for years, and we have developed strong social relationships not only in face-to-face situations but through social media as well. Face it. We are experts! Or are we? When it comes to intentional conversations with people, do you know how to craft a conversation in a way that encourages the other person to feel free to express his or her viewpoint? Can you craft a conversation to build a trusting relationship and establish honest interest in his or her well-being? Did you know that nurses use techniques to ensure people talk in lieu of one-word responses? Despite our insistence that we, as humans, intuitively know how to communicate, this chapter gives you a solid introduction into the art of communication in nursing practice—the art of therapeutic communication.

Therapeutic Communication: What Is It?

According to The *Free Medical Dictionary* (2020), therapeutic communication in health care refers to an interaction between a health care professional and a patient that aims to enhance the patient's comfort, safety, trust, or health and well-being" (para. 1).

This definition does not entirely encompass the true meaning or contextual application in nursing practice. As stated by Živanović and Ćirić (2017), therapeutic communication is defined as "a process in which the nurse consciously influences the patient or helps them in better understanding through verbal and nonverbal communication, while encouraging patients to express their feelings and ideas, which is an important prerequisite for the realization of relation of mutual acceptance and respect" (p. 2). In this way, therapeutic communication in nursing promotes personal growth and attainment of patients' health-related goals. This skill set is the key to the development and maintenance of all nurse-patient relationships. After all, communication is an essential component of working within an interdisciplinary health care team, it is the key to ensuring patient safety, and it is an established influence to improved patient satisfaction and clinical outcomes.

As a nurse, you communicate with patients and families to develop meaningful relationships. Within those relationships you collect relevant assessment data, provide education, and interact during nursing interventions. Conversations with patients and family members may seem social; however, no conversation with a nurse is ever without intent. Even when nurses are asking patients about their interests, they are collecting data to improve the nurse-patient relationship. Strong communication skills are the key to every nurse's ability to deliver patient-centered care.

Patient safety also requires effective communication among members of the health care team as patients move from one caregiver to another or from one care setting to another. Good communication skills help to reduce the risk of errors. Additionally, competency in communication maintains effective relationships within the entire sphere of professional practice and meets legal, ethical, and clinical standards of care.

Nursing Point of View

It is a well-known fact that nurses generally engage with patients over longer periods of time than other disciplines. In research published by Press Ganey (2020), a company that surveys patients about their care in inpatient settings, patients may feel more comfortable revealing information to nurses as nurses are at the bedside 70% more than any other discipline. This makes a nurse's ability to effectively and therapeutically communicate with a patient and family members absolutely essential. Additionally, nurses, by role, are involved in intimate physical acts such as bathing, feeding, and special procedures. As a result, patients and families may feel more comfortable in revealing information not always shared with physicians or other health care providers. Your ability to shape your care on the basis of this special knowledge provides an indispensable contribution to the overall care of your patient.

Talking with Patients and Developing the Nurse-Patient Relationship

Caring relationships are the foundation of clinical nursing practice; however, a therapeutic relationship promotes a psychological climate that facilitates positive change and growth.

Communication establishes caring, healing relationships.
The ability to relate to others is important for interpersonal communication.
Communication, including posture, expressions, gestures, words, and attitudes, has the power to hurt or heal.

The goals of a therapeutic relationship focus on a patient achieving optimal personal growth related to personal identity, ability to form relationships, and ability to satisfy needs and achieve personal goals. Patient's needs take priority over a nurse's needs. Your nonjudgmental acceptance of a patient is an important characteristic of the relationship as acceptance conveys a willingness to hear a message or acknowledge feelings. A caring relationship between the nurse and a patient does not just happen—the secret is revealed! Nurses create each relationship with skill and trust.

Think of the last time you engaged a friend or loved one in a conversation. Think about what you said and how you responded. Each sentence conveyed meaning and likely caused a reaction, whether positive or negative. That is because all behavior communicates and all communication influences behavior. Nurses with expertise in communication express caring by:

- Becoming sensitive to self and others.
- Promoting and accepting the expression of positive and negative feelings.
- Developing caring relationships.

- Instilling faith and hope.
- Promoting interpersonal teaching and learning.
- Providing a supportive environment.
- Assisting with gratification of human needs.
- Allowing for spiritual expression.

Relating to others includes the ability to take the initiative in establishing and maintaining communication, to be authentic (one's self), and to respond appropriately to the other person.

Effective interpersonal communication also requires a sense of mutuality (i.e., a belief that the nurse-patient relationship is a partnership and that both are equal participants). The Joint Commission (TJC) recognized the need to promote effective communication for patient- and family-centered care, cultural competence, and improved patient safety. Did you know that within health care facilities, this accreditation agency has initiated a set of standards for hospitals that promote these improvements in communication? Communicating effectively with patient and health care team members is critical to safe, effective care. Agencies such as TJC know that skilled communication empowers others to express what they believe and make their own choices; these are essential aspects of the individualized healing process.

Elements of Professional Communication

Appearance, demeanor, and behavior	Courtesy
Use of names	Trustworthiness
Autonomy and responsibility	Assertiveness

There are several essential elements of professional communication. These elements must first be in place before a nurse can employ therapeutic communication techniques. In addition, a professional is expected to be clean, neat, well groomed, conservatively dressed, and odor free. Patients and family members have very high expectations of nurses and the image created in the mind of people when they think about a nurse is equally challenged by the expectations of specific professional behaviors. This behavior reflects warmth, friendliness, confidence, and competence. Professionals speak in a clear, well-modulated voice; they use good grammar; they listen to others; they help and support colleagues; and most importantly, they communicate effectively. Think back to Chapter 3 in this text. What are the expected characteristics of a professional RN? Common courtesy is also a part of professional communication. To practice courtesy, begin exploring your ease with looking people in the eye, greeting people warmly and saying "hello" and "goodbye" to people as you meet with family and friends. In the patient care setting, nurses practice entering and exiting rooms, greeting people by using their formal title, and knocking before entering any private room or area. Professional appearance, demeanor, and behavior communicate that you have assumed the professional helping role, are clinically skilled, and are focused on your patients. Common courtesy is part of professional communication.

Always introduce yourself. Failure to give your name and status or to acknowledge a patient creates uncertainty about the interaction and conveys an impersonal lack of commitment or caring. To foster trust, communicate warmth and demonstrate consistency, reliability, honesty, competence, and respect.

Think back to our ethics section. Autonomy is being self-directed and independent in accomplishing goals and advocating for others. Professional nurses make choices and accept responsibility for the outcomes of their actions. Assertiveness allows you to express feelings and ideas without judging or hurting others. Assertive behavior includes intermittent eye contact; nonverbal communication that reflects interest, honesty, and active listening; spontaneous verbal responses with a confident voice; and culturally sensitive use of touch and space.

Developing Communication Skills

Gaining expertise in communication requires both understanding the communication process and reflection about one's communication experiences as a nurse. Nurses who develop critical thinking skills make the best communicators. They draw on theoretical knowledge about communication and integrate this knowledge with knowledge previously learned through personal clinical experience. They interpret messages received from others to obtain new information, correct misinformation, promote patient understanding, and assist with planning patient-centered care. When you consider a patient's problems, it is important to apply critical thinking and critical reasoning skills to improve communication in assessment and care of the patient. Perseverance and creativity are also helpful because they motivate a nurse to identify innovative solutions. Patients respond more readily to a nurse with a self-confident attitude. This is not the same as giving the impression of being arrogant. Nurses must be mindful of how they are perceived through the use of proper word choice, expression, and action. An attitude of humility is necessary to recognize when you need to better communicate and intervene with patients, especially when it is related to their cultural needs. Integrity allows nurses to recognize when their opinions conflict with those of their patients, review positions, and decide how to communicate to reach mutually beneficial decisions.

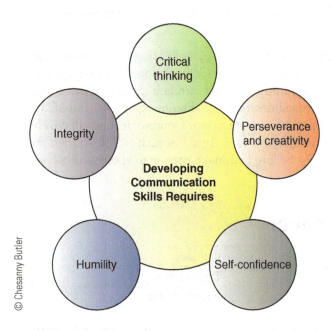

Perceptual Bias

What each person says is always influenced by perception. Perception can lead to bias. Perceptual bias is therefore defined as the tendency to form simplistic stereotypes and assumptions about something. Each individual bases his or her perceptions about information received through the five senses of sight, hearing, taste, touch, and smell. An individual's culture and education also influence perception. People often incorrectly assume that they understand an individual's culture. They tend to distort or ignore information that goes against their expectations, preconceptions, or stereotypes. Critical thinking helps nurses overcome perceptual biases or stereotypes that interfere with accurately perceiving and interpreting messages from others. Let's take a look at a video in which perception, bias, and behavior interpretation is explained using everyday context: https://study.com/academy/lesson/perception-bias-in-communication-within-organizations.html

By thinking critically about personal communication habits, you learn to control these tendencies and become more effective in interpersonal relationships. Nurses learn to integrate communication skills throughout the nursing process as you collaborate with patients and health care team members to achieve goals and to ensure safety.

The Communication Process

Communication is an ongoing and continuously changing process. You are changing, the people with whom you are communicating are changing, and your environment is also continually changing. This simple linear model represents a very complex process with its essential components. The circular transactional model includes several elements: the referent, sender and receiver, message, channels, context or environment in which the communication process occurs, feedback, and interpersonal variables. In this model, each person in the communication interaction is both a speaker and a listener and can be simultaneously sending and receiving messages. Both parties view the perceptions, attitudes, and potential reactions to a sent message. Feedback from the receiver or environment enables the communicators to correct or validate the communication. This model also describes the role relationship of the communicators as complementary and symmetrical. Complementary role relationships function with one person holding an elevated position over the other person. Symmetrical relationships are more equal.

The Components of Communication

The diagram on interpersonal variables represents the communication cycle which is initiated by a referent and influenced by interpersonal variables and the environment. The referent motivates one person to communicate with another. In a health care setting, sights, sounds, sensations, perceptions, and ideas are examples of cues that initiate the communication process. The sender is the person who encodes and delivers a message, and the receiver is the person who receives and decodes the message. The more the sender and the receiver have in common and the closer the relationship, the more likely they will accurately perceive one another's meaning and respond accordingly.

The message is the content of the communication. It contains verbal and nonverbal expressions of thoughts and feelings. Effective messages are clear, direct, and in understandable language.

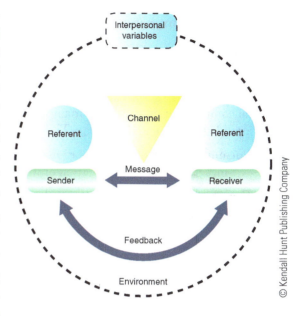

Communication channels are means of sending and receiving messages through visual, auditory, and tactile senses. Facial expressions send visual messages; spoken words travel through auditory channels. Touch uses tactile channels. Individuals usually understand a message more clearly when the sender uses more channels to send it. Feedback is the message a receiver receives from the sender. It indicates whether the receiver understood the meaning of the sender's message. Interpersonal variables are factors within both the sender and receiver that influence communication. Perception provides a uniquely personal view of reality formed by an individual's culture, expectations, and experiences. Each person senses, interprets, and understands events differently. The environment is the setting for sender-receiver interaction. An effective communication setting provides participants with physical and emotional comfort and safety.

Levels of Communication

There are five distinct levels or forms of communication. These levels involve the people, or an individual person/s involved in communication and represent unique styles that are effective in specific situations. These levels include: Intrapersonal, Interpersonal, Small group, Public, and Electronic contexts. *Intra*personal communication, also known as *self-talk*, is an individual's internal discussion when thinking. People's thoughts and inner communications strongly influence perceptions, feelings, behavior, and self-esteem. Nurses use intrapersonal communication when reflecting on a situation, assessing patients, and critically think through a process before communicating with others. *Inter*personal communication reflects a communication expression between two people. Notice that we are careful here not to say solely a verbal exchange as many people communicate with another using communication techniques. Think of this form of communication as an exchange of information with another person. Interpersonal communication requires a sender and receiver and the message that the receiver perceives may be quite different than what was intended. It is the level most frequently used in nursing situations and lies at the heart of nursing practice. Meaningful interpersonal communication results in an exchange of ideas, problem solving, and expression of feelings, decision making, goal accomplishment, team building, and personal growth. Small-group communication reflects communication within a group of people who usually come together because they share a common goal. This could be a support group, a research team, or a practice review committee. Generally, small group communication occurs with a manageable number of people who all know each other and are few in number so as to fit around a board table or form a circle of chairs in which each person can clearly observe, hear, and sense the communication of other group members. Public communication is interaction with an audience. Consider this type of communication as a format including a community presentation, a religious service, or other large group venue. People often do not know each other if it is a single event but gather for a common purpose such as a concert, a community town forum, academic course, or speech. Nurses often speak with groups of consumers about health-related topics, present scholarly work to colleagues at conferences, or lead classroom discussions with students.

Forms of Communication

There are three standard forms of communication, namely: verbal, nonverbal, and electronic.

Verbal Communication

Verbal communication comprises many components to ensure the communication process effectively conveys the intended message and meaning. These components include:

- **Vocabulary:** Verbal communication uses spoken or written words. Verbal language conveys specific meanings through the combination of words.

- **Denotative and connotative meaning:** Communication is unsuccessful if senders and receivers cannot translate one another's words and phrases. When you care for a patient who speaks another language, a professional interpreter is necessary. Limiting use of medical jargon to conversations with other health care team members improves communication. The connotative meaning is the shade or interpretation of the meaning of a word influenced by the thoughts, feelings, or ideas that people have about the word. You need to select words carefully, avoiding easily misinterpreted words, especially when explaining a patient's medical condition or therapy.

- **Clarity and brevity:** Conversation is more successful at an appropriate speed or pace. Speak slowly and enunciate clearly. Think before speaking, as long complex communication can be difficult to understand. Repeating important parts of a short concise message also clarifies communication.

- **Pacing:** Talking rapidly, using awkward pauses, or speaking slowly and deliberately conveys an unintended message. Long pauses and rapid shifts to another subject give the impression that you are hiding the truth.

- **Intonation:** Tone of voice dramatically affects the meaning of a message. Be aware of voice tone to avoid sending unintended messages. Effective communication is simple, brief, and direct.

- **Timing and relevance:** Timing is critical in communication. Even though a message is clear, poor timing prevents it from being effective. Patients report improved satisfaction, understanding, and perception of safety with registered nurses (RNs) who provided a bedside hand-off and communicate information about the plan of care.

Nonverbal Communication

Nonverbal communication includes the five senses and everything that does not involve the spoken or written word. Nonverbal communication is unconsciously motivated and more accurately indicates a person's intended meaning than spoken words. Because the meaning attached to nonverbal behavior is so subjective, it is imperative that you verify it.

- **Appearance**: Personal appearance includes physical characteristics, facial expression, and manner of dress and grooming. These factors communicate physical well-being, personality, social status, occupation, religion, culture, and self-concept.

- **Posture and Gait:** Body language, the way people choose to stand or hold themselves when talking and the manner or pattern in which a person walks are forms of self-expression.

The way people sit, stand, and move reflects attitudes, emotions, self-concept, and health status.

- **Facial Expressions, Eye Contact, and Gestures**: These convey emotions such as surprise, fear, anger, happiness, and sadness. Patients closely observe nurses; in fact, patients make their first assumptions about nurses within the first encounter by observing the way nurses walk, talk, and present themselves. Many people have a difficult time controlling their facial expressions when they encounter an unpleasant odor or injury. Although it is hard to control all facial expressions, try to avoid showing shock, disgust, dismay, or other distressing reactions in a patient's presence. Additionally, nurses should be very perceptive as people signal readiness to communicate through eye contact. Maintaining eye contact during conversation shows respect and willingness to listen but a lack of eye contact may indicate anxiety, defensiveness, discomfort, or lack of confidence in communicating. Gesturing can enhance verbal communication (such as a person who naturally talks with his or her hands or uses sign language as a primary method for communicating). Conversely, gestures can create their own unique or specific message which can be perceived positively or negatively (such as holding one fist straight up in the air in solidarity or waving at someone from across the room). Sounds such as sighs, moans, groans, or sobs also communicate feelings and thoughts. Combined with other nonverbal communication, sounds help to send clear messages.

Territoriality and Personal Space: A territory is a specific area that people mentally determine and claim as their own in a social setting. People often defend this area and perceive their temporary claim as a right to defined space, what is often meant by the expression, "I was here first." Have you not witnessed territoriality perhaps at a movie theater? How often have we been to a movie theater and noticed that within a select row of seats, a person has placed a coat or handbag in an empty seat so as to extend the distance between himself and a stranger. It represents a behavioral code for "I'm not comfortable being that close to a stranger and would like this to be my space." Territory is important because it provides people with a sense of identity, security, and control. Territoriality can be grouped into three distinct personal space violations: invasive looking (such as a person looking in a slightly cracked door of a patient room), invasive touch of person or possessions within the defined space, and invasive use of objects or equipment to both their personal space and or physical body. Personal space, as mentioned in the next section, involves the area or space around a person. A lack of awareness of how territoriality and personal space can impact a patient will result in a perceived threat by patients. Often nurses find that patients and family members act defensively in these instances which can be avoided by first acknowledging personal space, discussing appropriate distancing, and asking permission.

Electronic or Written Communication

Electronic communication is the newest category of communication but has become essential to health care communication in an ever-changing world. Electronic communication used to reflect how what we write in an e-mail is interpreted by those who read the information. This format of communication has definitely evolved to include multiple platforms of communication using technology. This could be social media, a patient portal for health care conversations with providers and the exchange of patient data, blogs, education feeds, or other modality that helps nurses form relationships with patients and their health care team.

Metacommunication

Metacommunication is a broad term that refers to all factors that influence communication. Awareness of influencing factors helps people better understand what is communicated.

Zones of Personal Space in Nursing Interaction

According to Marin, Gasparino, and Puggina (2018), the zones of personal space, although generally defined in distance between people, are most significantly influenced by a person's culture. The comfort with the distance between people has a great deal to do with the relationship formed between individuals, how a person perceives another, and what people are doing at the time of encounter. Within nursing, the intimate zone, although generally reserved for affectively close relationships, is the zone in which most procedures, assessments, and interventions must be performed. At this distance of immediate proximity to people, procedures may also require patients to be naked, placed in uncomfortable and private anatomic positions, or cause embarrassment

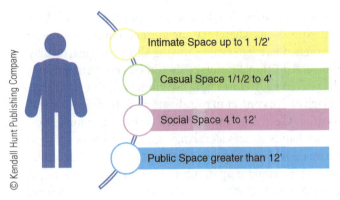

or nervousness. The role of the RN in these instances requires professional conduct and courtesy such as asking permission, ensuring a patient has a full understanding of the procedure or intervention and has time to process the encounter without surprise. Although seen by the nurse as a sign of attentiveness and care, sitting on the end of a patient's bed may represent a violation of intimate space for a person and cause him or her to become uncomfortable or nervous. Nurses must consider how they culturally understand appropriate personal space zones and work to understand that their own perceptions and parameters of comfort may not be shared by their patients. Nurses must always assess each situation and ask the patient for permission or guidance on what is acceptable in the nurse-patient relationship. Nurses frequently also use causal space zones with patients. You have probably noticed that when you go to the doctor's office and are placed in an examination room, the nurse or doctor engages you, either sitting or standing, at a reasonable distance, usually within 4 feet of your location. This is considered casual space. Placing a distance between the nurse and the patient allows people to comfortably exist in their own personal space without feeling a sense of space invasion. A general conversation is held within a casual space zone. This could be at a table in the library studying with friends or at dinner, it could also be a nurse standing at the side of a patient's bed or at the foot of the bed talking with a patient. Social space has never been more understood than during the pandemic crisis involving Covid-19. Social space requires a distance of generally 6 feet which offers room to engage in activities without feeling crowded but also permits audible conversation. The distance between a patient in a waiting area in a doctor's or dentist's office and the receptionist is generally 4 to 12 feet and is a great way to remember this zone. Finally, public space zones are used in nursing for presentations or lectures, conferences, and other large venue activities where the space between the nurse and perhaps the people being educated is greater than 12 feet.

Therapeutic Communication Techniques

Learning how to therapeutically communicate with others involves skill and repetition. In learning the following techniques, students are often asked to complete a process recording of a conversation that they have with an unsuspecting family member or friend. Process recordings help you practice the use of therapeutic techniques and analyze what was said unintentionally and/or revise what can be stated better in future conversations. The process recording is a written account of an interaction between a friend or family member and the student nurse. Through the reconstruction of the interaction the student is provided with an opportunity to retrospectively examine and analyze his/her communication skills, therapeutic use of self and the family member or friend's part in the interaction. The process recording is used to evaluate both participant's behaviors and approaches to therapeutic communication and effective communication.

The student nurse analyzes what is said (the content of the interaction) and the flow of the interaction (the process). This analysis augments the student nurse's ability to increase awareness of feelings, values, expectation, and assumptions. He or she is able to analyze verbal and nonverbal responses. In real life, process recordings help caregivers to distinguish between thoughts and feelings and find better ways to communicate more clearly and effectively.

The following represent therapeutic techniques for communicating with patients: Sharing observations, Sharing empathy, Sharing hope, Sharing humor, Sharing feelings, Using touch, Using silence, Providing information, Clarifying, Focusing, Paraphrasing, Validation, Asking relevant questions, Summarizing, Self-disclosure, Confrontation. Knowing how and when to use these techniques is part of the art of nursing communication and will become innate with practice. The following text provides examples of various positive or therapeutic communication techniques.

Using Broad Open-Ended Questions

The use of a broad opening statement allows the patient to set the direction of the conversation. Such questions as "Is there something you'd like to talk about?" give the patient an opportunity to begin expressing himself. In using a broad opening statement, the nurse focuses the conversation directly on the patient and communicates to him that she is interested in him and his problems. Upon sensing that the patient may have a need, the nurse can use a broad opening statement to initiate discussion, while at the same time allowing the patient to determine what will be discussed. When the patient opens the conversation, the nurse can then follow his lead to discover the meaning his opening remark had for him, encouraging him by question or comment to express himself further. Whether what he has said is of an obviously serious nature ("Am I dying"?), or less emotionally charged ("I'm going home tomorrow,") the nurse should avoid making assumptions as to its meaning or the need he may be expressing.

Using General Leads

During the conversation, general leads, such as "yes" or simply the "uh hum" will usually encourage the patient to continue. General leads, like broad opening statements, leave the direction of the conversation to the patient. They also convey to him that the nurse is listening and that she is interested in what he will say next. This can be accomplished verbally or nonverbally, by nodding or through facial expressions, which demonstrate attentiveness and concern. The major purposes of general leads is to encourage the patient to continue, and to speak spontaneously so that the nurse can learn from him how he perceives his situation, and get some idea of what his need may be. By becoming aware of and resisting any tendency she may have to jump to conclusions regarding the nature of the patient's problem, and instead of drawing him out, the nurse can begin to obtain the information she needs to be of continuing assistance to the patient. Some additional samples of general leads are: "I see." "And then….", "go on" and incomplete or open-minded sentences such as "You were saying that…"

Reflecting

In reflecting, all or part of the patient's statement is repeated to encourage him to go on. If he says, "Everyone here ignores me," the nurse might reply, "Ignores you?" Letting him hear all of what he has said, or part of what he has said may lead him to more fully consider and expand upon his remark. Reflecting can be overused, and the patient is likely to become annoyed if his own words or statements are continually repeated to him. Selective reflecting can be used once the nurse has begun to understand what the patient is driving at. For example, if the patient says, "I feel so tired, I don't like it here," the nurse can either reflect, "Tired?" or "You don't like it here," depending on which part of his statement she thinks is most important.

Sharing Observations

Here, the nurse shares with the patient her observations regarding behavior. The patient who has a need is often unaware of the source of this distress, or reluctant to communicate it verbally. However, the tension or anxiety created by his need creates energy which is transformed into some kind of behavior, nail biting, scratching, hand clenching, or general restlessness. By sharing her observations of this behavior with him, the nurse is inviting the patient to verify, correct, or elaborate on her observations. In doing so, she is attempting to find out from him the meaning of his behavior rather than assuming she knows. In her efforts to ascertain the meaning of the observed behavior, the nurse may share with the patient what he has actually perceived through her senses ("You are trembling"), or she may share her interpretation of what she has perceived ("You seem upset"). Generally, her perceptions tend to be correct; her interpretations of her perceptions, however, may often be incorrect. When sharing her observations of the patient's behavior, the nurse should phrase her remarks tentatively, in such a manner that it is her observation, rather than the patient's behavior which is being questioned. This observation can be accomplished by "afraid" or "angry" which may evoke a response of denial from the emotional impact, for example, "tense," "upset," or "restless."

Acknowledging the Patient's Feelings

The nurse helps the patient to know that his feelings are understood and accepted and encourages him to continue expressing them. If he were to say, "I hate it here. I wish I could go home," the nurse might respond, "It must be difficult to stay in a place you hate." When a patient talks about something that is upsetting to him or expresses a complaint or criticism, the nurse can convey acceptance by acknowledging the feelings he is expressing without agreeing or disagreeing with them. By sympathetically recognizing that it must be difficult or embarrassing or frightening or frustrating, and so on to feel as the patient does, she does not pass judgment on the thought or feeling itself. If communication is to be successful, it is essential that the nurse accept the thoughts and feelings her patient is expressing, irrespective of whether or not she, personally, thinks and feels the same way. For if the patient senses or is told that the nurse does not approve of or does not agree with what he is expressing, it is extremely unlikely that he will continue, or that a positive nurse-patient relationship will ensue.

Using Silence

In certain circumstances, an accepting, attentive silence may be preferable to a verbal response. This allows the nurse to temporarily slow the pace of the conversation and gives the patient an opportunity to reflect upon, and then speak further about his feelings. Also, silence allows the nurse to observe the patient for nonverbal clues and to assemble her own thoughts. Due to the nature of conventional social conversation, in which pauses and lulls are generally avoided, the nurse may instinctively become uneasy when the patient falls silent for any length of time. However, periods of silence are often most beneficial to the communication process allowing the patient to collect his thoughts and to reflect upon the topic being discussed. Maintaining an attentive, expectant silence at this time lets him know that his silence, too, is accepted. Because silence can convey much—sadness, distress, anger, contemplation—the nurse can also attempt to assess the meaning of the silence within the context of the conversation and with attention to accompanying nonverbal behavior. It is important to practice silence as the nurse tends to exaggerate the period of time a silence lasts due to her own anxiety. After several minutes of silence, the nurse can help the patient to resume verbal activity with statements such as, "You were saying that …" or "What were you thinking?"

Giving Information

Studies have shown that a major cause of anxiety or discomfort in hospitalized patients is lack of information or misconceptions about their condition, treatment, or hospital routines. When the patient is in need of information to relieve anxiety, form realistic conclusions, or make decisions, this need will often be revealed during the interaction by statements he makes. By providing such information as she prudently can, admitting and finding out what she does not know, or referring the patient to someone who can assist him, the nurse can do much to establish an atmosphere of helpfulness and trust in her relationship with the patient.

Clarifying

If the nurse has not understood the meaning of what the patient has said, she clarifies immediately. She can use such phrases as "I'm not sure I follow…" or "Are you using this word to mean…" to request that the patient make his meaning clear to her. In seeking immediate clarification when she is in doubt as to the patient's meaning, the nurse can prevent misunderstanding from hindering communication; also, because her efforts in clarifying will demonstrate her continued interest in what the patient is saying, the use of this technique can help motivate him to go on. Because meaningful communication depends greatly upon the extent to which the persons involved understand clearly what each has said, the nurse should not hesitate to interrupt the patient if there is any confusion in her mind about his meaning. She might say, "Before you go on, I want to understand what you meant by…" Also, the nurse should clarify identities, such as ambiguous "he" or "they." In addition, to enable the patient to best understand her, the nurse should avoid the use of medical terminology or jargon whenever possible and attempt to express herself in such manner appropriate to the patient's apparent level of understanding.

Verbalizing Implied Thoughts and Feelings

The nurse voices what the patient seems to have fairly obviously implied, rather than what he has actually said. For example, if a patient has said, "It's a waste of time to do these exercises" she might reply, "You feel they aren't benefiting you?" Besides, enabling the nurse to verify her impressions, verbalizing implied thoughts and feelings, the nurse should be careful to verbalize only what the patient has fairly obviously suggested so that she does not get into the area of offending interpretations—of making conscious that which is unconscious.

Exploring or Delving Further into a Subject or Idea

"Tell me more about that," "Would you describe it more fully?" and "What kind of work?" are examples exploring topics which the patient has brought up for discussion. The nurse should recognize when to delve further—she should refrain from probing or prying. If the patient chooses not to elaborate, the nurse should respect the patient's wishes. Probing usually occurs when the nurse introduces a topic because she is anxious.

Presenting Reality

Examples of presenting reality are: "I see no one else in the room," "That sound was a car backfiring," and "Your mother is not here; I'm a nurse." When it is obvious that the patient is misinterpreting reality, the nurse can indicate that which is real. She does this not by way of arguing with the patient or belittling his own experiences, but rather by calmly and quietly expressing her own perceptions or the facts in the situation. The intent here is merely to indicate an alternate line of thought for the patient to consider, not to "convince" the patient that he is in error. This technique is highly useful with patients who are confused and geriatric patients in nursing homes who show signs of confusion, psychiatric patients showing high anxiety, and patients who are confused due to alcohol or drugs such as LSD.

Voicing Doubt

Statements like the following express uncertainty as to the reality of the patient's perceptions: "Isn't that unusual?" "Really?" "That's hard to believe." Another means of responding to distortions of reality is to express doubt. Such expression permits the patient to become aware that others do not necessarily perceive events in the same way or draw the same conclusions that he does. This does not mean that he will alter this point of view, but at least he will be encouraged to reconsider and reevaluate what has occurred. And, the nurse has neither agreed nor disagreed, yet, at the same time, she has not let misinterpretations and distortions pass uncommented upon but rather suggesting collaboration by offering to share, to strive, to work together with the patient for his benefit.

"Perhaps you and I can discuss and discover what produces your anxiety (pain, frustration, etc.)." The nurse seeks to offer the patient a relationship in which he can identify his problems in living with others, grow emotionally, and improve his ability to form satisfying relationships with others. She offers to do things not for him or to him, but with him.

Validating

When the nurse feels that the patient's need has been met, she should validate her impression with him. If his reply to such a question as "Do you feel relaxed?" or "Are you feeling better now?" suggests his need has not been completely met, the nurse should renew her efforts to assist him. The nurse should not assume that she has been successful in meeting a patient's need until this has been validated with him. Also, since the patient may have needs in addition to that which the nurse has attempted to meet, validating gives him an opportunity to make any such needs known. Also, the nurse observes his nonverbal behavior. A lessening of tension or a positive change in behavior would support an affirmative verbal response; if tension or behavior is not perceptibly altered, however, an affirmative reply would not be as meaningful.

Using Observation

Nurses make observations by commenting on how the other person looks, sounds, or acts. Stating observations often helps a patient communicate without the need for extensive questioning, focusing, or clarification. For example, "I noticed that you cringe whenever someone begins to sing," is an example of using observation. This technique is generally followed by the use of an open-ended question such as "Can you tell me about that?" to allow the person to consider your observation and share his thoughts or feelings.

Sharing Empathy and Hope

Empathy is the ability to understand and accept another person's reality, accurately perceive feelings, and communicate this understanding to the other. Nurses recognize that hope is essential for healing and learn to communicate a "sense of possibility" to others. Appropriate encouragement and positive feedback are important in fostering hope and self-confidence and for helping people achieve their potential and reach their goals.

Using Humor

Humor is an important but often underused resource in nursing interactions. It is a coping strategy that can reduce anxiety and promote positive feelings. Patients use humor to release tension, cope with fear related to pain and suffering, communicate a fear or need, or cope with an uncomfortable or embarrassing situation. Emotions are subjective feelings that result from one's thoughts and perceptions. Feelings are not right, wrong, good, or bad, although they are pleasant or unpleasant. If individuals do not express feelings, stress and illness may worsen.

Using Appropriate Touch

Touch is one of the most potent and personal forms of communication. It expresses concern or caring to establish a feeling of connection and promote healing. Comfort touch such as holding a hand is especially important for vulnerable patients who are experiencing severe illness with its accompanying physical and emotional losses. Nurses need to be aware of patients' nonverbal cues and ask permission before touching them to ensure that touch is an acceptable way to provide comfort.

Using Silence

Silence prompts some people to talk. It allows a patient to think and gain insight. Remaining silent demonstrates patience and a willingness to wait for a response when the other person is unable to reply quickly. Sometimes techniques are artfully combined such as is the case when combining touch with silence. Over time nurses learn how and when to use techniques for different people based on their perceptual ability to understand a situation. Never attempt a technique without first watching an expert so that incorrect messages are not portrayed and alter the trust relationship with a patient.

Restating or Paraphrasing

Paraphrasing is restating another's message more briefly using one's own words. Through paraphrasing you send feedback that lets a patient know that he or she is actively involved in the search for understanding.

Providing Information

Providing relevant information tells other people what they need or want to know so they are able to make decisions, experience less anxiety, and they feel safe and secure. It is also an integral aspect of health teaching. To check whether you understand a message accurately, restate an unclear or ambiguous message to clarify the sender's meaning. In addition, ask the other person to rephrase it, explain further, or give an example of what the person means.

Using Focus

Focusing involves centering a conversation on key elements or concepts of a message. If conversation is vague or rambling or patients begin to repeat themselves, focusing is a useful technique because it helps the patient concentrate on what is important.

Validation

Validation is a technique that nurses use to recognize and acknowledge a patient's thoughts, feelings, and needs. Patients and families know they are being heard and taken seriously when the caregiver addresses their issues.

Asking Relevant Questions or Exploring

Nurses ask relevant questions to seek information that is needed for decision making. Ask only one question at a time and fully explore one topic before moving to another area. Use both open-ended and closed-ended questions. Asking too many questions is sometimes dehumanizing.

Summarizing

Summarizing is a concise review of key aspects of an interaction. It brings a sense of satisfaction and closure to an individual conversation and is especially helpful during the termination phase of a nurse-patient relationship.

Self-disclosure

Self-disclosures are subjectively true personal experiences about the self that are intentionally revealed to another person. This is not therapy for a nurse; rather it shows a patient that the nurse understands his experiences and that they are not unique.

Gentle Confrontation

When you confront someone in a therapeutic way, you help the other person become more aware of inconsistencies in his or her feelings, attitudes, beliefs, and behaviors.

Nontherapeutic Communication Techniques

Certain communication techniques hinder or damage professional relationships. These specific techniques are referred to as *nontherapeutic* or *blocking* and often cause recipients to activate defenses to avoid being hurt or negatively affected. Asking personal questions that are not relevant to a situation simply to satisfy your curiosity is not appropriate professional communication. When a nurse gives a personal opinion, it takes decision making away from the other person. It inhibits spontaneity, stalls problem solving, and creates doubt. Changing the subject when another person is trying to communicate his or her story is rude and shows a lack of empathy. It blocks further communication, and the sender then withholds important messages or fails to openly express feelings. Perceptual bias or stereotypes are generalized beliefs held about people. Making stereotypical remarks about others reflects poor nursing judgment and threatens nurse-patient or team relationships. When a patient is looking for understanding, false reassurance discourages open communication. Offering reassurance not supported by facts or based in reality does more harm than good. Sympathy is concern, sorrow, or pity felt for another person. A nurse often takes on a patient's problems as if they were his or her own. Some nurses are tempted to ask patients why they believe, feel, or act in a certain way. Regardless of a patient's perception of your motivation, asking "why" questions causes resentment, insecurity, and mistrust. It is important that nurses not impose personal attitudes, values, beliefs, and moral standards on others while in the professional helping role. Other people have the right to be themselves and make their own decisions. Judgmental responses often contain terms such as *should, ought, good, bad, right,* or *wrong*. Becoming defensive in the face of criticism implies that the other person has no right to an opinion. The sender's concerns are ignored when the nurse focuses on the need for self-defense, defense of the health care team, or defense of others. Passive responses serve to avoid conflict or sidestep issues. They reflect feelings of sadness, depression, anxiety, powerlessness, and hopelessness. Aggressive responses provoke confrontation at the other person's expense. They reflect feelings of anger, frustration, resentment, and stress. Challenging or arguing against perceptions denies that they are real and valid. Therapeutic communication seems so challenging when we break it down and analyze what we say and how we can be more responsive and effective care providers. Over time, student nurses learn these skills and are able to appropriately and professionally communicate therapeutically with patients in a way that seems natural and social. Like any skill, this takes time and repetition.

The following techniques represent what "not" to do when attempting to therapeutically engage another person in a conversation. Examples for each technique are also provided as context. Often, we find that without training, many of the following techniques are used in communicating with others, especially when we do not know what to say, how to handle a situation, find silence awkward, or perceive that what we are saying is helpful when it is not.

Using Reassuring Clichés

"Everything will be all right," "You don't need to worry," "You're doing fine," are reassuring clichés which are often given automatically or may be used when a person has difficulty knowing what to say. Although the nurse may say, "Everything will be all right," out of a sincere desire to reduce the patient's anxiety, such a response may also result from an unrecognized need to reduce her own anxiety to feel more comfortable herself. When a patient who has expressed apprehension is told, "Everything will be alright," he is likely to feel that the nurse is not interested in his problem and thus will refrain from discussing it further. Reassuring clichés tend to contradict the patient's perception of his situation, thus implying that his point of view is incorrect or unimportant. When there are facts that are reassuring, the nurse can give genuine reassurance by communicating them to the patient. A less direct but basic reassurance is given as the nurse communicates to the patient understanding, acceptance, interest.

Giving Advice

"What you should do is…" "Why don't you…?" By telling the patient what he should do, the nurse imposes her own opinions and solutions on his, rather than helping him to explore his ideas so that he can arrive at his own conclusions. Even when a patient clearly asks for advice, the nurse should be cautious in her response, and supply only pertinent information that may give him a better basis for decision making. Giving the patient advice may imply to him that the nurse thinks she knows what is best for him, and that she feels his problem can be easily solved. If the patient does not accept these implications, he may resent the nurse for advising him, if he does accept them, it may reinforce his feelings of dependency. If, instead of giving advice, the nurse helps the patient to think through and attempt to resolve his problems for himself, she makes an important contribution to his feelings and self-esteem. When a patient asks for advice, the nurse can assist him by asking such questions as "Tell me what your feelings are about…" She can provide pertinent information (facts, resource people, services, etc.) and help him examine all parts of the problem by encouraging him to express his own thoughts and feelings about the problem and helping him to identify possible solutions and the factors involved in possible outcomes. While it is obvious that some patients, by reason of age or extreme physical or emotional stress are incapable of this kind of activity, the nurse should foster decision making to whatever extent is possible.

Giving Approval

"That's the right attitude," or "That's the thing to do." Although conceivably a useful response when the nurse wishes to motivate or encourage a patient, giving approval can sometimes create a block by shifting the focus of the discussion to the nurse's values or feelings, and by implying standards of what is and what is not acceptable.

The nurse's approval of a patient's statement such as "I know I shouldn't let it get me down," makes it difficult for him to admit that it is getting him down. Approval also implies that the nurse's concepts of right and wrong will be used in judging the patient's behavior. For it is possible that the nurse may approve behavior of which the patient himself disapproved—such as crying or expressing strong feelings. In such cases, the values and goals of the nurse would conflict with those of the patient. To the extent then that (1) a standard has been set that the patient may not at another time be able to achieve, (2) a value judgment has been given and the patient may be consciously or subconsciously aware that nonacceptance of at least some type of behavior has been implied, (3) that the patient may be motivated to repeat the behavior for the sake of approval, rather than because he himself values the results, (4) that the focus of the conversation is on the nurse's values of goals rather than the patient's, and (5) that the patient may not value or may disapprove those actions or expressed feelings of which the nurse approved—to this extent giving approval may function to block communication.

Requesting an Explanation

"Why did you do that?" "Why are you here?" "Why are you upset?" are examples of questions which some patients find difficult and even intimidating because they call for the patient to immediately analyze and explain his feelings or actions. Patients who cannot answer "why" questions frequently invent answers. The nurse should avoid asking "why" questions except when asking simple, direct questions pertaining to patient care, for example, "Why are you going to the bathroom?" In general, the nurse is of more assistance, however, if she assists the patient to describe his feelings. There are two types of questions the nurse can ask in order to get descriptive information: closed and open questions. A closed question is phrased so that a yes or no answer is indicated, for example, "Did you sleep well last night?" or so that a specific choice of answers is given within the questions, for example, "Do you want this injection in your right or left arms?" Although this type of question does not encourage the patient to express himself or give him the lead, it can be useful in eliciting specific information that is needed to assist the patient once his need has been identified. It is also useful in caring for the patient who has limited energy or who by reason of age or severe stress is mentally or emotionally incapacitated. Open questions, though still determined by the subject, let the patient provide his own answers. Words such as "who," "what," "when," and "where" elicit factual information and will help the patient to begin learning to describe his experiences. "How" questions should usually be avoided also since they ask by what process or for what reasons; some patients will respond to "How do you feel?" with my fingers.

Agreeing with the Patient

"I agree with you," or "You must be right." "When the nurse introduces her own opinions or values into the conversation, it can prevent the patient from expressing himself freely. By agreeing with the patient she can make it difficult for him to later change or modify the opinion he has stated. Or, if he has expressed something other than what he actually believes to be true (sometimes to test the nurse to see if she's interested in him) he may be prevented from saying what he really thinks at a later time. Rather than stating her own views, the nurse should accept the patient's statements and encourage him to elaborate on them by using responses such as general leads or reflecting.

Expressing Disapproval

"You should stop worrying like this," or "You shouldn't do that." When the nurse indicates that she disapproves of the patient's feelings or actions, she imposes her own values, rather than accepting the patient's. Such negative value judgment may intimidate or anger the patient and will often block communication by expressing disapproval; the nurse implies that she is entitled to make negative value judgments regarding his behavior, and that he is expected to conform to her standards. If the patient accepts this role, communication will probably be hindered as he modifies his behavior to avoid incurring further disapproval. Rather than making value judgments about a patient's behavior, the nurse can encourage further examination of a remark with statements such as "You feel that…" or "You seem to be…"

Belittling the Patient's Feelings

"I know just how you feel," "Everyone gets depressed at times." Because the patient is usually primarily concerned with himself and his own problems, telling him that others have experienced or are experiencing the same feelings will seldom do much to comfort him. On the contrary, to do so devalues his feelings, implying that his discomfort is commonplace and insignificant. The nurse can communicate understanding, acceptance, and interest in him as an individual by simply acknowledging his feelings. "This must be very difficult (upsetting, exhausting, annoying, etc.) for you."

Disagreeing with the Patient

"You're wrong," "That's not true," "No, it isn't." By contradicting the patient, the nurse indicates to him that what he has said has not been accepted. Because the nurse's judgment may cause him to feel threatened, he may refrain from expressing himself further on the subject, or he may become defensive or angry. When the patient makes a statement with which the nurse disagrees, she can acknowledge his feelings and opinions without agreeing with them, for example, "Then you feel…" or "I hear what you are saying."

Defending

"Your doctor is quite capable." "She's a very good nurse." In defending herself, others, or the hospital in response to criticism from a patient, the nurse not only communicates a nonaccepting attitude to him, but also, in becoming defensive, may lead to believe that his criticism is justified. Thus, this response may reinforce rather than change the patient's point of view. By acknowledging the patient's feelings, without agreeing or disagreeing—for example, "It must be difficult for you to feel this way"—the nurse avoids putting herself in opposition to the patient.

Making Stereotyped Comments

"How are you feeling?" "Isn't it a beautiful day?" "It's for your own good," "You'll be home in no time." By using social clichés or trite phrases, the nurse may lead the patient to reply in a like manner, thus keeping the conversation at a superficial level. While comments such as "How are you feeling?" may be used purposefully to elicit information, they are often made automatically, or out of a subconscious desire to avoid uncomfortable topics. In addition to social clichés she already uses, the nurse in her daily work may develop or adopt "stock" replies which she used in her interactions with patients. Because they are easy to use, they are a convenient substitute for a more thought-out and individualized response. They may also be used when the nurse is unsure of an answer to a patient's question, and she is reluctant to admit that she does not have the answer. When the nurse has nothing meaningful to say, she should remain silent. Social clichés and stock replies function to keep distance between the nurse and the patient. Behind stereotyped responses, there may be stereotyped attitudes on the part of the nurse.

Changing the Patient's Subject

"I'd like to die," Nurse: "Don't you have visitors this weekend?" or "By the way…" or "That reminds me…." Generally, the nurse changes the subject to avoid discussing a topic which makes her uncomfortable (consciously or unconsciously) or to initiate discussion of a topic in which she is more interested. In either case, by taking the lead in the conversation away from the patient, she can block any attempt he may be making to express his needs to her. Even when he is discussing a matter that seems to be of relatively little significance, the nurse may be able to pick up clues that will help identify his needs, or the patient may be proceeding in a roundabout way toward making his needs known.

Giving Literal Response to a Patient

"They're looking in my head with a TV." Nurse: "What channel?" or Patient: "That doctor is a pain in the neck." Nurse: "Would you like your pain medication?" Patients who are confused or highly anxious may have difficulty describing their experiences. They may use words in a very personal sense which has meaning to them but can be misinterpreted by the nurse. If the nurse responds to his comment as if it were a statement of fact, she tells the patient she cannot understand when anxiety-producing feelings are being described. Instead, she could respond with, "Tell me what it means to you." or "I'd like to understand that better; tell me more."

Challenging

"If you're dead, why is your heart beating?" "Your sister couldn't be coming, she's dead." Often the nurse feels that if she can challenge the patient to prove his unrealistic ideas he will realize he has no proof. She forgets that the patient's ideas and perceptions serve a purpose for him, that they conceal feelings and meet needs that are real. When challenged, the patient tends only to strengthen and expand his misinterpretations as he seeks support for his point of view. Rather than challenging the patient's views, the nurse might restate, or ask him to "say more about that" so she can understand the patient's viewpoint more clearly.

Adapting Communication Techniques

Caring for patients with communication barriers may include the use of alternative therapeutic communication techniques through various modes. These patients may include patients who cannot speak clearly (meaning they have had some kind of expression impairment), people who have experienced a cognitive impairment, people who have a hearing impairment, people who have a visual impairment, people who are unresponsive, or even people who do not speak English (or your language) as a primary form of communication. Interacting with people who have conditions that impair communication (visual, hearing) requires special thought and sensitivity. Such patients benefit greatly when you adapt communication techniques to their unique circumstances, developmental level, or cognitive and sensory deficits. A nurse directs actions toward meeting the goals and expected outcomes identified in the plan of care, addressing both the communication impairment and its contributing factors. Effective communication involves adapting special needs resulting from sensory, motor, or cognitive impairments. This is often the case when caring for older adults who have lost partial sensory abilities due to disease or the process of aging. With older adults it is important to encourage them to share life stories and reminisce about the past because such socialization has a therapeutic effect and increases their sense of well-being. Patients with impaired verbal communication require special consideration and alterations in communication techniques to facilitate sending, receiving, and interpreting messages. As such, The National League for Nursing (NLN) has an exceptional web page directed solely at communicating with people with disabilities: http://www.nln.org/professional-development-programs/teaching-resources/ace-d/additional-resources/communicating-with-people-with-disabilities

Their platform, notably ACED or Advancing Care Excellence for Persons with Disabilities, is a significant resource for care providers interested in learning how to properly adapt and effectively use communication techniques for people with numerous disabilities. Persons with disabilities of any kind will find standard communication ineffective and thus the care we provide substandard. Failure of nurses to provide proper accommodations for communication is a major barrier to safe, effective care and highly unethical. Imagine for a moment being visually impaired and having someone shout at you. Too often people respond in nontherapeutic ways when faced with situations in which they are not trained or find competence. Ensuring that each nurse has the proper clinical experience and academic preparation for caring for people with any form of disability is an essential standard of care. How can nurses best make these adjustments to communication when we know that personal space, visual cues, and basic patient interactions are highly visual? Additionally, patients who may primarily or solely speak another language are unable to understand nurses and providers who speak English. Imagine for a moment needing to seek medical care in a foreign country and not being able to understand a single word anyone would be saying to you. Would you trust what people were doing if you did not know their culture or practices? Would you be alright with people giving you medications without anyone telling you what the medication was or what it is being used for? It is unacceptable in today's world to not use an approved medical interpreter or interpreter device for translation. A national standard of practice for interpreters in health care and a code of ethics were both developed to guide the level of quality required to provide interpreter services for medical purposes. These standards are regulated by the National Council on Interpreting in Health Care and can be accessed here: https://www.ncihc.org/assets/documents/publications/NCIHC%20National%20Standards%20of%20Practice.pdf

In nursing and medical ethics, it is a patient's right to access health care in a means that is fully comprehensible in their preferred language (Basu, Phillips-Costa, & Jain, 2017). This is especially important when considering significant legal implications such as informed consent with medical procedures or surgeries.

Interprofessional Teamwork

While taking a class, many times students are asked to work in groups. In fact, within an introduction to professional nursing class, many assignments and in-class activities involve group work. Yet, as a student, a general distaste for group work prevails. Why do people not like to work with others? Is it that people find it simply easier to work alone? Is group work inconvenient? Or, is it that people find it difficult to manage teams because there is limited communication and discussion of expectations? Working in teams requires planning, scheduling, and consideration of other people? Teamwork requires a different kind of work relationship. Working in a group requires specific behaviors and competencies that are often not well developed in professional fields. Because of this, when people are required to work in groups, they bemoan the experience and generally do their best to tolerate it. Think back in your life. Have you ever received training in how to properly cooperate with another person, exchange information in a professional way, or understand the individual roles of other fields of study? Most people can say that they have not and yet, teamwork is often an essential component of most careers. In nursing and health care, teamwork is essential. Nurses must work well in health care teams, every single day, on behalf of their patients. Nurses need the expertise of other disciplines in health care to ensure the best possible outcome. While nurses work in tandem with health care providers, such as physicians and nurse practitioners, other essential services are often consulted for specific concerns. Teams of people from various disciplines come together and hold what are referred to as *case conferences* to ensure all dimensions of the patient are considered in the management of care. With patient care conditions being extremely complex, there is a need for special care and expertise from many fields. These teams could include physicians, nurses, specialists, nutritionists, case managers, social workers, and chaplains just to name a few. Additionally, disciplines come together to train inpatient care situations. Consider practicing patient care emergencies. Would it be more effective to train realistically involving all the members of the health care team or individually by discipline? When it comes to emergencies such as a cardiac arrest or the resuscitation of a newborn, it is imperative that nurses know how to effectively work with other disciplines so that care is streamlined, expectations and roles are clarified, and care becomes timely and highly effective. In academia, many universities recognize the value of learning and training in interprofessional contexts and intentionally host interprofessional courses to ensure teamwork competencies are learned from the beginning and students learn to rely on, trust, and value the exchange of viewpoint and ideas of different fields of study.

Quality and Safety Education for Nurses (QSEN) has developed a series of competency training modules. One of the most important is the competency training focused on learning Teamwork and Collaboration. Take a moment to watch and review the module below so that you become familiar with the three key components of teamwork and collaboration in nursing practice. You will be asked to create an account using the login credentials: AACNQSEN. Use the credentials provided for both the login User ID and Password. You will be able to create your own personal account so that you can take advantage of their other learning modules at a later time: https://presentations.icohere.com/IC/AACN-QSEN/Disch-TC18/presentation_html5.html

Interprofessional Collaboration Behaviors

When working together in a team, on behalf of a patient or family, it is essential that all team members understand the group dynamic rules. Similar to establishing class rules on the first day of an academic course, team members must all understand the behaviors that are expected from one another when engaging in interprofessional collaborative opportunities. These behaviors, as established by the Interprofessional Professionalism Collaborative (2016) include the ability for highly effective communication, respect for each other's view point/contributions and belief systems, altruism and caring (meaning each team member values placing the needs and concerns of the patient ahead of his own and conducts himself with concern for the welfare of the patient), excellence in providing and expecting only the highest quality of care, ethics and individual as well as team professional accountability. Knowing what the expectations are of any group, as well as understanding what training and competence is expected, helps each team member trust and value all contributions.

IPEC Competencies

The Interprofessional Education Collaborative (IPEC) developed core competencies for interprofessional collaborative practice in 2016 (IPEC, 2016). Within this foundational document, IPEC provides the following key definitions:

> **Operational Definitions Interprofessional education:** "When students from two or more professions learn about, from and with each other to enable effective collaboration and improve health outcomes" (WHO, 2010).
>
> **Interprofessional collaborative practice:** "When multiple health workers from different professional backgrounds work together with patients, families, [careers], and communities to deliver the highest quality of care" (WHO, 2010).
>
> **Interprofessional teamwork:** The levels of cooperation, coordination, and collaboration characterizing the relationships between professions in delivering patient-centered care. **Interprofessional team-based care:** Care delivered by intentionally created, usually relatively small work groups in health care who are recognized by others as well as by themselves as having a collective identity and shared responsibility for a patient or group of patients (e.g., rapid response team, palliative care team, primary care team, and operating room team).
>
> **Professional competencies in health care:** Integrated enactment of knowledge, skills, values, and attitudes that define the areas of work of a particular health profession applied in specific care contexts.
>
> **Interprofessional competencies in health care:** Integrated enactment of knowledge, skills, values, and attitudes that define working together across the professions, with other health care workers, and with patients, along with families and communities, as appropriate to improve health outcomes in specific care contexts (p. 8).

IPEC Core Competencies 2016:

https://learn-us-east-1-prod-fleet01-xythos.s3.amazonaws.com/5dd6acf5e22a7/11674205?response-cache-control=private%2C%20max-age%3D21600&response-content-disposition=inline%3B%20filename%2A%3DUTF-8%27%27IPEC%2520Core%2520Competencies%25202016.pdf&response-

Interprofessional Collaboration Competency Domains

These four interprofessional collaboration competencies reflect the dimensions of the ANA Standards of practice for professional nursing as well as the Code of Ethics discussed earlier in this text. Each of the following competencies are subsequently broken down into sub competencies for greater understanding.

Chapter 6 Patient and Health Team Communication

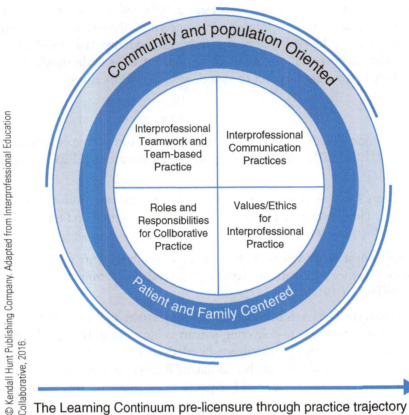

The Learning Continuum pre-licensure through practice trajectory

© Kendall Hunt Publishing Company. Adapted from Interprofessional Education Collaborative, 2016.

Competency 1
Work with individual of other professions to maintain a climate of mutual respect and shared values. (Values/Ethics for interprofessional Practice)

Competency 2
Use the knowledge of one's own role and those of other professions to approximately assess and address the health care needs **of patients** and **to Promote and advance the health of populations.** (Roles/Responsibilites)

Competency 3
Communicate with patients, families, communities, **and professionals in health and other fields** in a responsive and responsible manner that supports a team approach to the **promotion and** maintenance of health and the **prevention and** treatemnt of disease. (Interprofessional Communication)

Competency 4
Apply relationship-building values and the principles of team dynamics to perform effectively in different team roles to **plan, deliver, and evaluate** patient/poulation-centered care **and population health programs and policies** that are safe, timely, efficient, effective, and equitable. (Teams and Teamwork)

Summary

Nurses must remember their listening skills as a key component of nursing practice, not only as a therapeutic strategy with patients but also as a standard of professional daily practice with other health care team members. Nurses must practice active listening and be aware of nonverbal cues, display honesty and courtesy, provide empathy, and work to ensure the messages provided to peers, administrators, physicians, and other health care team members reflect the clarity and brevity required in effective communication. While this chapter seeks to introduce the student to the concepts of interprofessional communication and collaboration, communication will be an important thread that you will learn across any nursing program curriculum.

References

Basu, G., Phillips-Costa, V., & Jain, P. (2017). Clinicians' obligations to use qualified medical interpreters when caring for patients with limited English proficiency. *AMA Journal of Ethics, 19*(3), 245–252. doi:10.1001/journalofethics.2017.19.3.ecas2-1703. Retrieved from https://journalofethics.ama-assn.org/article/clinicians-obligations-use-qualified-medical-interpreters-when-caring-patients-limited-english/2017-03

Interprofessional Education Collaborative. (2016). *Core competencies for interprofessional collaborative practice: 2016 update*. Washington, DC: Author. Retrieved from https://learn-us-east-1-prod-fleet01-xythos.s3.amazonaws.com/5dd6acf5e22a7/11674205?response-cache-control=private%2C%20max-age%3D21600&response-content-disposition=inline%3B%20filename%2A%3DUTF-8%27%27IPEC%2520Core%2520Competencies%25202016.pdf&response-content-type=application%2Fpdf&X-Amz-Algorithm=AWS4-HMAC-SHA256&X-Amz-Date=20200608T120000Z&X-Amz-SignedHeaders=host&X-Amz-Expires=21600&X-Amz-Credential=AKIAZH6WM4PLTYPZRQMY%2F20200608%2Fus-east-1%2Fs3%2Faws4_request&X-Amz-Signature=fd3dd1a90e3724563346b06b4b77274d390231930f013d391ad4c643eb676cd9

Interprofessional Professionalism Collaborative. (2016). *Interprofessional professionalism behaviors*. Alexandria, VA: Author. Retrieved from http://www.interprofessionalprofessionalism.org/

Marin, C. R., Gasparino, R. C., & Puggina, A. C. (2018). The perception of territory and personal space invasion among hospitalized patients. *PloS One, 13*(6), e0198989. Retrieved from https://doi.org/10.1371/journal.pone.0198989

Press Ganey. (2020). *Nursing special report: The far-reaching impact of nursing excellence*. Retrieved from http://images.healthcare.pressganey.com/Web/PressGaneyAssociatesInc/%7B980c39eb-7cf2-4e71-8be4-694149ee8768%7D_2020_PG_Nursing_Special_Report.pdf

World Health Organization. (2010). *Framework for action on interprofessional education & collaborative practice*. Geneva, Switzerland: Author.

Živanović, D., & Ćirić, Z. (2017). Therapeutic communication in health care. *SciFed Nursing & Healthcare Journal, 1*(2), 1–7. Retrieved from https://www.researchgate.net/publication/320245946_Therapeutic_Communication_in_Health_Care

Chapter 7

Health Literacy

Chapter Objectives

- What is health literacy and how is it different than basic literacy?
- Why is health literacy important in nursing?
- How would a nurse use health literacy to engage in effective patient education?

What Is Health Literacy?

The Patient Protection and Affordable Care Act of 2010, Title V, defines health literacy as:

> the degree to which an individual has the capacity to obtain, communicate, process, and understand basic health information and services to make appropriate health decisions (Sec 5002 Definitions, p. 518).

Basically, it is the ability to understand and use health information correctly. Health literacy includes numeracy skills or the ability to use numbers and solve problems in day-to-day activities.

A person's ability to calculate his blood sugar levels, ability to properly measure medications or understanding nutrition labels are all skills requiring math application in day-to-day activities. Choosing between health plans or comparing prescription drug coverage requires calculating premiums, copays, and deductibles. In addition to basic literacy skills, health literacy requires knowledge of health topics. People with limited health literacy often lack knowledge or have misinformation about the body as well as the nature and causes of disease. Without this knowledge, they may not understand the relationship between lifestyle factors such as diet and exercise and various health outcomes. Health information can overwhelm even persons with intermediate literacy skills. What people may have learned about health or biology during their school years often becomes outdated or it is incomplete. Moreover, health information provided in a stressful or unfamiliar situation is often forgotten.

While current definitions of health literacy are from *Healthy People 2030*, The Association of University Centers on Disabilities (AUCD) and other monitoring agencies, specifically identify a wide range of skills paramount to improving health literacy levels. These skills have now become part of extensive community outreach programs in an attempt to significantly improve American health literacy levels.

How Is It Different Than Basic Literacy?

What is basic literacy? Kirsch (2001) as noted in the Institute of Medicine's 2004 report entitled, *Health Literacy: A Prescription To End Confusion*, defines basic literacy as "a person's ability to read, write, speak, and compute and solve problems at levels necessary to: (1) Function on the job and in society, (2) Achieve one's goals, and (3) Develop one's knowledge and potential" (Institute of Medicine, Committee on Health Literacy;

Nielsen-Bohlman, Panzer, & Kindig, 2004, p. 335). The term *illiteracy* means being unable to read or write. A person who has limited or low literacy skills is not illiterate and may not have low basic literacy skills at all. In fact, a significant number of those who studied in the NAAL (2003) as discussed in the following text have low health literacy despite above average basic literacy. So why is this happening in our society?

Health Literacy Importance

The U.S. Department of Education administered a National Assessment of Adult Literacy (NAAL) in 2003 to obtain a baseline of health literacy levels in the United States. In this project, the Department of Education chose to report these data based on four levels of health literacy. These levels included below basic, basic, intermediate, and proficient.

According to Kutner, Greenberg, Jin, Boyle, Hsu, and Dunleavy (2007),

> Below basic literacy level is described as no more than the most simple and concrete literacy skills and demonstrates an extreme inability to navigate healthcare processes and education. Basic literacy level refers to skills necessary to perform simple and everyday literacy activities, giving those in this category the ability to interpret only the simplest of healthcare information and process. Intermediate literacy level encompasses skills necessary to perform moderately challenging literacy activities, containing individuals who can moderately navigate healthcare education and processes and make correct inferences. Proficient literacy refers to skills necessary to perform more complex and challenging literacy activities which includes people who can read, write and understand complex healthcare education and processes. (p. 8)

Of interest, 53% of those included in the study demonstrated an intermediate level of health literacy, or roughly half. Very few (12%) participants had a proficient level of health literacy, the level at which a person could easily navigate health care resources and information. The subsequent level outcomes were as follows: basic health literacy 22%; below basic 14%. These statistics should cause nurses to pause and reflect on the difficulty that a significant number of patients encounter in understanding patient education, making appointments, adhering to medication directions, and navigating insurance. In total, a shocking 36% of participants in the NAAL or one-third of the study population, had basic or below basic health literacy skills. (Kutner, Greenberg, Jin, & Paulsen, 2006). As reported in *The Health Literacy of America's Adults: Results From the 2003 National Assessment of Adult Literacy* report from 2006, "low health literacy has been linked to poor health outcomes (higher rates of hospitalization and less frequent use of preventive services). Both of these outcomes are associated with higher healthcare costs" (Cuddahee, 2016, para 2).

Nursing Implications

Let's watch and learn from Lisa Fitzpatrick, a public health expert from St Louis Missouri, who gave a TED talk in 2016 on the impact of health literacy in the United States. As you watch this presentation, can you relate to her findings? Do you have difficulty with health care information? What can be done? Access the following URL to learn more: https://youtu.be/-x6DLqtaK2g

In a report from the Joint Commission (2007) entitled, *What Did the Doctor/Nurse Say? Improving Health Literacy to Protect Patient Safety*, the most frequently noted safety issue connected to limited health literacy is the risk of medication errors that result from improper dosing administration when patients are at home. In addition, low health literacy is significantly related to poorer understanding of medication names, indications, and instructions as well as adherence to treatment plans. Patients are also less likely to engage in making health care appointments timely when faced with the common difficulties attributed to access and health care insurance rules and regulations. This is a critical finding as nurses need to know at what level to educate patients correctly and how well they understand their own health insurance coverage so that patients and families can be empowered to participate in care.

How Can Nurses Help People with Low Health Literacy?

If the nurse is unable to quickly use a health literacy assessment tool, as discussed later in this chapter, to determine a person's current level of health literacy, the nurse should assume that the person may have difficulty understanding all of the instructions provided. In this case, our role is to help all patients who need health information and services. To do this we must be abreast of all current community resources and know how and where to refer a patient. We must know whom to communicate with on behalf of a patient within the health care team or network. Nurses often find, print, and explain health information data as well as schedule appointments and services so that we know that the patient will maintain a continuity of care. Nurses may work with social workers and other community resource agents to help patients communicate needs and preferences, provide repetition in education, and/or alternate formats of information so that the patient can process small manageable pieces of health data easily. Nurses may also work with patients and their families to decide which information and services match the needs and preferences of the patient so health information and services can be effective and timely.

Those at Risk

Populations most likely to experience low health literacy are:

- older adults,
- racial and ethnic minorities,
- people with less than a high school degree or GED certificate,
- people with low income levels,
- non-native speakers of English,
- and people with compromised health status

Education, language, culture, access to resources, and age are all factors that affect a person's health literacy skills (Cuddahee, 2016, para 3).

Health literacy is important for everyone because, at some point in everyone's life, people need to be able to find, understand, and use health information and services. Taking care of personal health is part of everyday life, not just when people visit a doctor, clinic, or hospital. Health literacy can help prevent health problems and protect health, as well as better manage unexpected emergencies. Even people who read well and are comfortable using numbers can face health literacy issues when:

- They are not familiar with medical terms or how their bodies work.
- They have to interpret statistics and evaluate risks and benefits that affect their health and safety.
- They are diagnosed with a serious illness and are scared and confused.
- They have health conditions that require complicated self-care.
- They are voting on an issue affecting the community's health and relying on unfamiliar technical information.

Active Learning Activity:

Use the following interactive Health Literacy Data Map sponsored by the University of North Carolina at Chapel Hill to look at current health literacy levels in your area. The map can be accessed using the following link: http://healthliteracymap.unc.edu

What can we tell about health literacy by looking at a map? Notice that there is a correlation between impoverished areas and low health literacy levels. What else can we see using the data map? Notice that there are also significantly low levels of health literacy in affluent areas as well. Why is this? Health literacy does not equate with general literacy or necessarily with education level and can be found in all neighborhoods and at all economic levels. Nurses encounter patients every day who are very well educated and are, in fact, at the top of their fields, but they have difficulty understanding medical instructions, navigating insurance processes, and require assistance in interpreting directions for medications.

Health Literacy Assessment Tools

The Health Literacy Tool Shed funded by the U.S. National Libraries of Medicine is a repository of more than 200 global health literacy assessment tools. Offered in multiple languages, the tools provided offer both specific medical condition health literacy tools and tools for general health literacy assessment. See https://healthliteracy.bu.edu/all.

In addition, The Agency for Healthcare Research and Quality Health Literacy also houses a complete database of the most common and reliable health literacy assessment tools. See: https://www.ahrq.gov/topics/health-literacy.html. The repository also offers access to professional education and training, patient education resources, and published papers.

One of the most reliable (α 0.89) and quick general health literacy tools is known as the *Short Assessment of Health Literacy or SAHL-S&E*, provided in both English and Spanish. Used with adults aged 18 to 64, this face-to-face assessment tool contains only 18 items providing medical word associations to general language contexts. The tool is simple and effective, providing two scoring categories. The person administering the SAHL should write the stem word at the top of a notecard and the Key or distracter words under the stem so as to show all 3 words to the viewer for each of the 18-word combinations below. If the score on the tool is between 0 and 14, the person being assessed has an inadequate health literacy level sufficient for managing their health in today's world. The SAHL-S&E assessment tool and user guides for both the English and Spanish versions can be found as a pdf here: https://www.ahrq.gov/health-literacy/quality-resources/tools/literacy/index.html.

SAHL-E Word Sets & User's Guide

Stem	Key or Distracter		Don't know
1. kidney	__urine	__fever	__don't know
2. occupation	__work	__education	__don't know
3. medication	__instrument	__treatment	__don't know
4. nutrition	__healthy	__soda	__don't know
5. miscarriage	__loss	__marriage	__don't know
6. infection	__plant	__virus	__don't know
7. alcoholism	__addiction	__recreation	__don't know
8. pregnancy	__birth	__childhood	__don't know
9. seizure	__dizzy	__calm	__don't know
10. dose	__sleep	__amount	__don't know
11. hormones	__growth	__harmony	__don't know
12. abnormal	__different	__similar	__don't know
13. directed	__instruction	__decision	__don't know
14. nerves	__bored	__anxiety	__don't know
15. constipation	__blocked	__loose	__don't know
16. diagnosis	__evaluation	__recovery	__don't know
17. hemorrhoids	__veins	__heart	__don't know
18. syphilis	__contraception	__condom	__don't know

Directions to the Interviewer:
Before the test, the interviewer should say to the examinee:

> *"I'm going to show you cards with 3 words on them. First, I'd like you to read the top word out loud. Next, I'll read the two words underneath and I'd like you to tell me which of the two words is more similar to or has a closer association with the top word. If you don't know, please say 'I don't know'. Don't guess."*

Show the examinee the first card.

The interviewer should say to the examinee:

> *"Now, please, read the top word out loud."*

The interviewer should have a clipboard with a score sheet to record the examinee's answers. The clipboard should be held such that the examinee cannot see or be distracted by the scoring procedure.

The interviewer will then read the key and distracter (the two words at the bottom of the card) and then say:

> *"Which of the two words is most similar to the top word? If you don't know the answer, please say 'I don't know'."*

The interviewer may repeat the instructions so that the examinee feels comfortable with the procedure.

Continue the test with the rest of the cards.

A correct answer for each test item is determined by both correct pronunciation and accurate association. Each correct answer gets one point. Once the test is completed, the interviewer should tally the total points to generate the *SAHL-E* score.

A score between 0 and 14 suggests the examinee has low health literacy.

The primary researcher for the development of the SAHL-S&E invites your questions and provides the following contact information:

Shoou-Yih Lee
Email: sylee@umich.edu
Department of Health Management and Policy
The University of Michigan School of Public Health
1415 Washington Heights, Ann Arbor, MI, 48109-2029

Summary

In this chapter, health literacy and its importance to nursing and patient care were identified. The essential difference between health literacy and basic literacy revealed that people who are well educated frequently have low health literacy scores. This information should inform the student learner with the tools needed to determine the ease and comfort a patient may have with health information. By assessing each patient, accurate health education and improved continuity of care can be provided to patients and their families.

References

Cuddahee, J. (2016). *Health literacy is a growing problem for all Americans*. Retrieved from https://www.literacynewyork.org/news/article/current/2016/10/10/100005/health-literacy-is-a-growing-problem-for-all-americans

Institute of Medicine, Committee on Health Literacy; Nielsen-Bohlman, L., Panzer, A. M., & Kindig, D. A. (Eds.). (2004). What is health literacy? In *Health literacy: A prescription to end confusion* (Chapter 2). Washington, DC: National Academies Press. Retrieved from https://www.ncbi.nlm.nih.gov/books/NBK216035/

Kirsch, I. S. (2001). The framework used in developing and interpreting the International Adult Literacy Survey (IALS). *European Journal of Psychology of Education, 16*(3), 335–361.

Kutner, M., Greenberg, E., Jin, Y., & Paulsen, C. (2006). *The health literacy of America's adults: Results from the 2003 National Assessment of Adult Literacy.* Washington, DC: U.S. Department of Education and National Center for Education Statistics. Retrieved from http://nces.ed.gov/pubsearch/pubsinfo.asp?pubid=2006483

Kutner, M., Greenberg, E., Jin, Y., Boyle, B., Hsu, Y.-C., & Dunleavy, E. (2007). *Literacy in everyday life: Results from the 2003 National Assessment of Adult Literacy.* Retrieved from https://nces.ed.gov/Pubs2007/2007480.pdf

Patient Protection and Affordable Care Act, V, U.S.C. § 5002 p. 581 (2010). Retrieved from http://housedocs.house.gov/energycommerce/ppacacon.pdf

Chapter 8

Introduction to Medical Abbreviations

Chapter Objectives:

- Define abbreviation.
- Determine why abbreviations are used in health care.
- Identify the potential problems when using abbreviations in nursing practice.

According to *Merriam-Webster* (2020), an abbreviation is defined as "a shortened form of a written word or phrase used in place of the whole word or phrase." Within the context of the English language used in the United States, our everyday speech and electronic communication is often filled with shortened expressions. Found in the *Urban Dictionary*, as provided by JasLeo (2018), the following abbreviations are commonly used in texting. Used in a textual reference, abbreviations in this way might resemble the following statement: Hey Jo, **WYD**? Your **SO** just posted a **PIC** of **U** from the party. **PPL** are **LOL** but **IDC RLY**, I think it's great. **TB L8R**, my **PITR**.

IDK—I don't know	PIC—Picture	L8R—Later
IDC—I don't care	WYD—What you doing	BTW—By the way
RLY—Really	U—You	IDK—I don't know
LOL—Laughing out loud	JK—Just kidding	BFF—Best friends forever
SO—Significant other	PPL—People	BTW—By the way
NVM—Never mind	TBH—To be honest	ROFL—Rolling on the floor laughing
M8—Mate	Ly2—Love you too	PAW—Parents are watching
TB—Text back	LyL—Love you loads	PITR-Parents in the room

Using abbreviations therefore represents a shorter, easier way to communicate not only in today's world but throughout history. The difficulty is that if you do not understand what the abbreviations mean, it becomes very difficult to communicate in this way. An important message or statement might be misinterpreted. While this might not be necessarily harmful in casual conversation, imagine the consequences within a field like health care, if providers, nurses, and other team members did not understand what was being written. The reason that abbreviations are used in health care setting, therefore, is not to ensure we have our own secret language but rather to provide us with a way that can save time while charting, taking notes, or giving report. While many medical records today are electronic, some facilities continue to use paper charting methods and records. Abbreviations in this instance also provide a mechanism to save space when documenting narrative entries. Let us review some common abbreviations you may have seen on signs in a hospital or medical center, on health care worker badges, in a medication prescription, or written within a medical note or set of forms to be filled out at the doctor's office. In addition to abbreviations, nurses use acronyms and medical terminology to accurately describe, define, and document health information. Once again, just like with the abbreviations and acronyms of common urban language and texting, it is important to understand the context and direct meaning of what is being used to ensure accurate interpretation.

LPN—Licensed Practical Nurse	DOB—Date of Birth	Hx—History
RN—Registered Nurse	PRN—When required	H&P—History and physical
ER—Emergency room	DVT—Deep vein thrombosis	HA—Headache
CPR—Cardiopulmonary Resuscitation	BP—Blood pressure	YO—Year old
DNR—Do not resuscitate	C/O—Complaint of	N/V—Nausea and vomiting
LMP—Last menstrual period	D/C—Discharge	SOB—Shortness of breath
F/U—Follow up	PMH—Past medical history	MVA—Motor vehicle accident

Here is an example. See if you can read the following medical statement using the reference box above. Ms. Smith is a 47 **YO** female **C/O HA** and **N/V** × 7 days. Her **PMH** reveals an **MVA** one week ago. At that time, she presented to the **ER** but was **D/C'd** without complication and urged to **F/U** to her primary physician.

In this chapter, you will learn the most common and basic abbreviations that are used in health care to help you build a foundation for reading and writing health care information. In addition, we will discuss the inherent flaws or problems with the use of abbreviations which led to the creation of a very specific "Do Not Use" list, by the Joint Commission (2019), to ensure patient safety and decrease confusion of interpretation.

Common Abbreviations Used in Health Care

See the following list of common medical abbreviations. These abbreviations should be memorized and learned in such a way that the nursing student can not only recite their meaning but also apply the abbreviations in context as demonstrated in the earlier example. The student nurses will use these abbreviations daily, throughout their entire nursing career. Use the flashcard generator associated with this textbook to guide you in this learning process.

ac	before meals	pc	after meals	ad lib	as desired
bid	twice a day	tid	three times a day	po	by mouth
prn	when required, as needed	qam	every morning	qpm	every night
qhs	daily at hour of sleep	qd	daily	qh	every hour
q2h	every 2 hours	q3h	every three hours	q4h	every four hours
qid	four times a day	qod	every other day	NPO	nothing per oral
OTC	over the counter	D/C	discharge	BP	blood pressure
c̄	with	p̄	after	s̄	without
ā	before	gtt	drop	t	teaspoon
T	tablespoon	tab	tablet	cap	capsule
os	mouth	hs	hour of sleep	HS	half strength
ADL	activities of daily living	ak-	above the knee	bk-	below the knee
ap/lat	anterior/posterior and laterally	Dx	diagnosis	Hx	history
Sx	symptoms	BM	bowel movement	DOB	date of birth
f/u	follow up	R/T	related to	RRR	regular rate and rhythm
BCP	birth control pills	LOC	level of consciousness	NKA	no known allergies

NKDA	no known drug allergies	ROM	range of motion	ROS	review of systems
DTR	deep tendon reflex	EENT	eyes ears nose throat	ENT	eyes nose throat
EKG	electrocardiogram	EEG	electroencephalogram	PERRLA	pupils equal round reactive to light and accommodation
PMH	past medical history	SL	sublingual	subQ	subcutaneous
IM	intramuscular	ID	intradermal	IV	intravenous
IVPB	intravenous piggyback	stat	immediately	UA	urinalysis
UTI	urinary tract infection	URI	upper respiratory infection	bs	blood sugar
CHD	coronary heart disease	CV	cardiovascular	CVA	cardiovascular accident
MI	myocardial infarction	CHF	congestive heart failure	CPR	cardiopulmonary resuscitation
MVA	motor vehicle accident	H&P	history and physical	R/O	rule out
LMP	last menstrual period	HTN	hypertension	BPH	benign prostatic hyperplasia
DVT	deep vein thrombosis	GERD	gastroesophageal reflux disease	GI	gastrointestinal
GU	genitourinary	GYN	gynecol-ogy/-ogic	N/V	nausea and vomiting
HA	headache	KUB	kidneys ureters and bladder	Lat	lateral
LLE	left lower extremity	LLL	left lower lobe	LLQ	left lower quadrant
LML	left medial lobe	LUE	left upper extremity	LUL	left upper lobe
LUQ	left upper quadrant	RLE	right lower extremity	RLL	right lower lobe
RLQ	right lower quadrant	RML	right medial lobe	ABG	arterial blood gas
ABO	blood group systems	DNR	do not resuscitate	NS	0.9 normal saline
½ NS	0.45 normal saline	LR	lactated ringers	D5LR	5% dextrose in lactated ringers
D5 1/2NS	5% dextrose in .45 normal saline	bpm	beats per minute	HOB	head of bed
I & O	intake and output	KVO	keep vein open	KUB	kidney, ureter, and bladder
TCDB	turn, cough, deep, breathe	GERD	gastroesophageal reflux disease	HCG	human chorionic gonadotropin hormone
UGI	upper gastrointestinal	AS	left ear	HDL	high density protein
AU	both ears	OD	right eye	LDL	low density lipoprotein
OU	each eye or both eyes	OS	left eye	CT	Computer axial tomography
AD	right ear	Rx	prescription	MRI	magnetic resonance imaging
CHF	congestive heart failure	COPD	chronic obstructive pulmonary disease	IDDM	insulin dependent diabetes mellitus
CSF	cerebrospinal fluid	CNS	central nervous system	gr	grains (unit of measure)
IBS	irritable bowel disease	PTSD	posttraumatic stress disorder	PPD	purified protein derivative
ASAP	as soon as possible	ASA	medication abbreviation for aspirin	O2	oxygen
CO2	carbon dioxide	AFIB	atrial fibrillation	ECHO	echocardiogram
CBC	complete blood count (lab test)	CBR	complete bed rest	BR c̄ BRP	bedrest with bathroom privileges
BSA	body surface area	LP	lumbar puncture	C/O	complaint of

For an exhaustive list of medical abbreviations used in health care, see F. A. Davis Taber's Online Medical Abbreviations (Venes, 2017).

Abbreviations No Longer Recommended

The Joint Commission is an independent, nonprofit agency that accredits health care organizations in the United States. The goal of the agency is to develop and uphold standards that impact quality patient care and safety in the health care industry. Have you ever heard of the Good Housekeeping seal of approval? This seal represents an iconic American designation which stems from the early 1900s. The Good Housekeeping Seal on a product packaging identifies the product as one that has undergone rigorous independent evaluation by scientists and engineers and that has been found to be highly reliable, safe, and effective, in keeping with the product company's claims. In health care, the Joint Commission puts health care facilities through a similar concept of rigorous examination to ensure health facilities provide safe and effective care practices that are in the best interest of the public and supported by the latest evidence-based practice and research. In lieu of a "seal," facilities passing their rigorous review earn what is called "accreditation." The Joint Commission also develops new standards based on data surrounding the health and safety of patient care. In 2001, the Joint Commission issued an alert to the public and health care industry involving the topic of the unsafe use of medical abbreviations. Subsequently, a National Patient Safety Goal was created requiring accredited health care organizations to restrict the use of certain abbreviations to avoid potential medical documentation, interpretation, and transcription errors for patient safety. The official "Do Not Use" list is provided below with permission from the Joint Commission (2019).

Official "Do Not Use" List

- This list is part of the Information Management standards
- Does not apply to preprogrammed health information technology systems (i.e. electronic medical records or CPOE systems), but remains under consideration for the future

Organizations contemplating introduction or upgrade of such systems should strive to eliminate the use of dangerous abbreviations, acronyms, symbols and dose designations from the software.

Official "Do Not Use" List

Do Not Use	Potential Problem	Use Instead
U, u (unit)	Mistaken for "o" (zero), the number "4" (four) or "cc"	Write "unit"
IU (International Unit)	Mistaken for IV (intravenous) or the number 10 (ten)	Write "International Unit"
Q.D., QD, q.d., qd (daily)	Mistaken for each other	Write "daily"
Q.O.D., QOD, q.o.d, qod (every other day)	Period after the Q mistaken for "I" and the "O" mistaken for "I"	Write "every other day"
Trailing zero (X.0 mg)* Lack of leading zero (.X mg)	Decimal point is missed	Write X mg Write 0.X mg
MS	Can mean morphine sulfate or magnesium sulfate	Write "morphine sulfate" Write "magnesium sulfate"
MSO₄ and MgSO₄	Confused for one another	

¹ Applies to all orders and all medication-related documentation that is handwritten (including free-text computer entry) or on pre-printed forms.

*Exception: A "trailing zero" may be used only where required to demonstrate the level of precision of the value being reported, such as for laboratory results, imaging studies that report size of lesions, or catheter/tube sizes. It may not be used in medication orders or other medication-related documentation.

Development of the "Do Not Use" List
In 2001, The Joint Commission issued a *Sentinel Event Alert* on the subject of medical abbreviations. A year later, its Board of Commissioners approved a National Patient Safety Goal requiring accredited organizations to develop and implement a list of abbreviations not to use. In 2004, The Joint Commission created its "Do Not Use" List to meet that goal. In 2010, NPSG.02.02.01 was integrated into the Information Management standards as elements of performance 2 and 3 under IM.02.02.01.

6/19

©2019 The Joint Commission | May be copied and distributed | Department of Corporate Communications

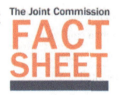

The Joint Commission

FACT SHEET

For more information

- Contact the Standards Interpretation Group at 630-792-5900.
- Complete the Standards Online Question Submission Form.

Official "Do Not Use" List from the Joint Commission

In comparing the previous medical abbreviations found in the *Common Abbreviations Used in Healthcare* section, with the "Do Not Use" list provided to the left, you will note several abbreviations that are no longer recommended for use. As with many skills and processes in health care, it is imperative that you familiarize yourself with the meaning of all abbreviations so that you can reduce your potential for error in not only interpretation but in documentation within your own nursing practice. Let me give you a related example. With the creation of electronic blood pressure machines, one might consider that there would be no reason to learn the complexity and accurate selection, application, and techniques involved in taking a manual blood pressure. Why go to all of the trouble of learning the complexity of doing something by hand or old school when you can use a machine to take the blood pressure? The answer is that not all facilities provide electronic blood pressure machines; in fact, as a nurse, you will work in many settings, homes, and even foreign countries that do not possess such a thing. Additionally, there are a few conditions in which the accuracy of an electronic blood pressure reading cannot be compared with the accuracy of taking the blood pressure manually. What if the machine fails or is no longer operational? Would you simply tell your patient, "Sorry, I can't take care of you today." A statement such as this related to training incompetence would never be acceptable to any patient needing care. In nursing we must always learn the proper way of doing everything to ensure we have competency in all situations, and at all times.

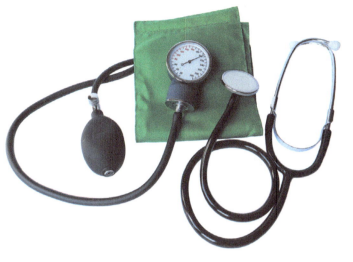

© MrVettore/Shutterstock.com

For this same reason, nurses must learn abbreviations and systems of measurement that may be rarely seen or practiced. The potential of their use in current practice, despite safety guidelines, will happen and nurses must know what to do and how to interpret these data.

Standards Regarding Abbreviations and Safe Patient Care

The Joint Commission standards, involved in the accreditation process, form the foundation of their evaluation process which in turn helps organizations set goals, measure, and improve patient quality and safety outcomes. The 4th standard in the accreditation of hospitals identifies that hospitals will use standardized diagnostic terms and procedure codes, and approved symbols and abbreviations in the care of the patient (The Joint Commission, 2020). This document reflects the common errors seen in health care that directly impact patient care. Look carefully at the document—not only does it reflect the abbreviation that should not be used in clinical practice, but it also clarifies the potential problem and presents the alternative. Additionally, this document prohibits the use of abbreviations in any document that a patient or family member must read and understand. That should make sense as we discussed how abbreviations have to be learned in order to be understood. The general public is not exposed to medical abbreviations in a way that would ensure comprehension. Recall our health literacy chapter ensuring that patients and family members are always assessed for health literacy and provided with the most clear and concise information possible. Within the hospital setting important documents such as informed consent for procedures and surgeries, patient right acknowledgements, discharge instructions should never contain abbreviations. In addition, standardizing abbreviations, both with regard to what not to use and what can safely be implemented improves the communication and understanding between all health care workers which leads to safe and efficient patient care. The "Do Not Use" list also discusses the safe use of periods and training zeros when writing out numbers, especially as it applies to medication orders. In Chapters 10 and 11 we will discuss safety, specifically as it relates to patient care and the accuracy of writing and interpreting medial orders and medications.

Practice Resource 1

In this exercise, practice interpreting the following medical order for nursing care. For each entry, rewrite the order, using the meaning for each abbreviation in the corresponding blank. If you misinterpret the abbreviation, what impact would it have on patient care?

Order	Meaning
Example: VS q shift and prn, report T>101F	Vital signs every shift and as needed. Report a temperature of greater than 101 ° F.
Activity: CBR	
TCDB q2h and prn	
Monitor I&O	
Diet: NPO	
Radiology: STAT portable CXR, PA& LAT	
Tylenol 325mg 2 tabs po Q4H prn discomfort	
Patient may take personal OTC medications	
Ancef 1gm IVPB now and then Q8h x 3 doses	

Answers:

Order	Meaning
Example: VS q shift and prn, report T>101F	Vital signs every shift and as needed. Report a temperature of greater than 101 °F.
Activity: CBR	Complete bed rest
TCDB q2h and prn	Turn, cough, and deep breathe every 2 hours as needed
Monitor I&O	Monitor intake and output
Diet: NPO	Nothing per oral
Radiology: STAT portable CXR, PA& LAT	Immediately obtain a portable chest x-ray with anterior/posterior as well as lateral views
Tylenol 325mg 2 tabs po Q4H prn discomfort	Give two 325mg Tylenol tablets every 4 hours as needed for discomfort
Patient may take personal OTC medications	Over the counter
Ancef 1gm IVPB now and then Q8h x 3 doses	Give Ancef 1 gram intravenous piggyback now and every 8 hours for 3 doses

Practice Resource 2

Student Medical Abbreviation Practice Quiz

Do you feel you have a good understanding of medical abbreviations to include tests, procedure, diseases, and language used in patient care delivery? Try the free medical abbreviations contextual quiz to test your skill by Health Information Technology Notifications (hitnots) found here: https://hitnots.com/medical-abbreviations-quiz/.

Like most, medical abbreviations are new and will require constant study and addition to ensure competency. After studying the lists provided in this chapter, try the following 30 question quiz to continue practice.

Summary

In nursing and health care, hundreds of standardized abbreviations exist and are used in basic care practices every day. Learning these abbreviations and their safe use improves not only a nurse's ability to interpret care orders but also to quickly record information needed for patient care. In nursing school, it is the role of the student to memorize these abbreviations and begin using them in clinical practice. Equally important is the understanding of safety and quality regulatory agency data and the creation of lists that contain abbreviations that should no longer be used in practice. Understanding these differences and working toward exceptional patient safety in all aspects of professional nursing is paramount.

References

The Joint Commission. (2019). *Official "do not use" list*. Retrieved from https://www.jointcommission.org/-/media/tjc/documents/resources/patient-safety-topics/do_not_use_list_6_28_19.pdf

The Joint Commission. (2020). *2020 comprehensive accreditation manual for hospitals* (1st ed.). Oak Brook, IL: Joint Commission Resources.

Merriam-Webster.com. (2020). Abbreviation [definition]. Retrieved from https://www.merriam-webster.com/dictionary/abbreviation

Venes, D. (Ed.). (2017). *Taber's medical dictionary* (23rd ed.). Philadelphia, PA: F. A. Davis. Retrieved from https://www.tabers.com/tabersonline/view/Tabers-Dictionary/767492/all/Medical_Abbreviations

Chapter 9

Introduction to Medical Terminology

Chapter Objectives:

- Describe why the use of medical terminology is important in health care.
- Identify the basic components of medical terms.
- List common tricks and devices used in learning medical terminology.
- Memorize prefix, root, and suffix components as a means of figuring out the meaning of each medical word.
- Pronounce, define, and spell each medical term correctly.

Medical terminology is the standardized means of communication within the health care industry. The importance of fluency in medical terminology, which applies to all hospital personnel, including allied health care professionals, cannot be overstated. Your role as a student nurse requires that you have a solid foundation in medical terminology in order to be successful in your coursework and in your clinical role. Medical terminology standardizes the description of body part, system, describes the body location, and patient symptoms. Using a standardized language enables everyone involved in the process of treatment and care to perform more efficiently for the patient's benefit. As we learned in the previous chapter, medical terminology contains numerous abbreviations and understanding them makes documentation much faster and easier. Although it seems a bit intimidating at first glance, medical terminology is not difficult. The majority of terms are derived from Greek and Latin. The science-based vocabulary follows a systematic methodology; each term contains two or three components and can be broken down into parts. Once you discover how the prefix, root, and suffix work together to generate meaning you will be well on your way to easily reading, writing, and interpreting medical words used in everyday practice. In this chapter we will also discuss basic anatomy, physiology, pathology, and diagnostic testing that is common in health care. As you are aware, the prerequisites to any nursing program are heavily based in the sciences. Your ability to break words into their basic components will help you succeed in both anatomy and physiology as well as pathophysiology course work. The best way to learn medical terminology is to become familiar with the structure and the most commonly used components. Let us begin with the basic components of medical terms.

Basic Components of Medical Terms

According to Chabner (2015), most medical terms consist of five basic components: root word (the base of the term, can be one or more), prefixes (letter groups in front of the root word, not all medical words have a prefix), the combining vowel (vowel that links the root to the suffix or root to root), the combining form (the combination formed from the root and the combining vowel together), and the suffix (letter groups at the end of the root word, all medical words have a suffix). When placed together, these components define a particular medical term. As most words do not easily fit together, a combining vowel, such as an "o" is often used as the link or glue between the components of the word. The combining vowel does not have a meaning by itself, it simply represents the connection. Understand the definition through common root words, prefixes, and suffixes. Recognizing these can greatly enhance memorization because it will help you define terms by applying the meaning of the prefixes/suffixes with the root word. For example, the term *carditis* contains the root word *card* which refers to the heart, and the suffix *itis*, which means inflammation. By knowing these two terms independently, we can conclude that it refers to inflammation of the heart. The term *subpulmonic* means "situated under the lung base" and refers to the location of fluid, what is called an *effusion* that can be seen on an x-ray between the base of the lung and the diaphragm. This word is an example of a medical term involving all three components.

Sub is the prefix meaning *below or under*. The word root pulmonary means *lung* and the suffix -ic means *pertaining to*.

Tips, Tricks, and Devices for Learning Medical Terminology

First, it is important that the learner does not attempt to simply memorize the words. Instead, think about what you are really being asked to do: learning terms using the divided components. The second important concept is to always link the word to the body part of the system and/or its function. This is important because some medical terms have specific context or meaning related to the body part. The third critical component of learning medical terminology is to make sure you can correctly pronounce and spell each word. Pronouncing a word incorrectly and spelling a word incorrectly can have devastating effects on patient care leading to error and clinical misinterpretation.

Three General Rules

There are basic rules to learning terminology properly. The first thing that should be done is to look at the suffix. The suffix provides you with the meaning. Then move backward. This is recommended because it allows you to spot the combining vowel if the letter before the suffix is an "a, e, i, o, or u." There are two additional components usually found in each word: the combining form (the root word plus the combining vowel) and the prefix. Although many medical words do not have a prefix, it is important to identify it properly, if one is present, because a prefix can change or influence the meaning by itself.

Once again, the trick to learning words is simple if you follow these three actions: (1) *Read*, (2) *Drop*, and (3) *Keep*. *Read* the meaning of the medical word from the suffix back to the beginning of the term. Second, *drop* the combining vowel (in most cases it is an "o" before a suffix that begins with a vowel; here is an example, carditis, not cardioitis. Third, *keep* the combining vowel between two roots in any word; for example, gastroenterology, not gastroenterology.

Tip # 1

Medical terminology is usually taught by body system, so for each system make flash cards that can help you study. Write the medical term on the front of the card and its definition on the back or if you prefer making electronic flashcards, use the flashcard maker associated with this text to help you. Flashcards quickly help you determine what you do not know. When you look at a particular term, you can guess the definition and then check if it is correct. If you prefer an app for your phone, Brainscape is a free mobile and online flashcard app that will easily convert your words into flashcards.

Tip #2

The end goal is to get to a point where you will not have to check if you are correct. This repetitive study method will help you learn the medical terminology through visualization.

Using the medical dictionary will enrich your vocabulary and deepen your understanding of the meanings and use of medical terms. You can buy access to medical terminology apps for your phone or you can access the *Oxford Concise Medical Dictionary* (8th ed.) for free using the following link:

https://www.oxfordreference.com/view/10.1093/acref/9780199557141.001.0001/acref-9780199557141?btog=chap&hide=true&pageSize=20&skipEditions=true&sort=titlesort&source=%2F10.1093%2Facref%2F9780199557141.001.0001%2Facref-9780199557141

Tip #3

Look up each new word and see what language it comes from and how it is pronounced. Many free online dictionaries have a pronunciation feature. You can always ask your professor to say the terms out loud to help you clarify pronunciation as well.

Tip #4

An organized list of items is easier to memorize than an unorganized list. If possible, group or categorize medical terminology based on a commonality. For example, you may group anatomical terms with the respective system of the body they may be associated with.

Be an active learner, and not a passive one. This means you need to have initiative. Rather than simply reading and writing the terms, apply them actively throughout the day by: discussing the definitions with others (classmates, friends), using the terms in a sentence on your own and with others, and teaching the terms to others.

Tip #5

There is a variety of games and quizzes that can help you learn medical terminology through practice. They also introduce a little fun to (otherwise) tiring theoretical learning. Multiple choice, memory, and matching games are a perfect fit when trying to learn terminology. You will be able to access practice resources at the end of this chapter that offer fun alternatives for learning the medical terminology essential to competent nursing practice.

Let's begin now by becoming familiar with common prefixes used in medical words. The following table provides the information you are required to know for nursing school.

Prefixes	Meaning
a-, an-	no, not, without
ab-	away from
ad-	toward
ana-	up, apart
ante-	before, forward
anti-	against
auto-	self, own
bi-	two
brady-	slow
cata-	down
con-	with, together
contra-	against, opposite
de-	down, lack of
dia-	through, complete
dys-	bad, painful, difficult, abnormal
ec-	out, outside
en-, endo-	in, within
epi-	upon, on, above
eu-	good, normal

(continued)

Prefixes	Meaning
ex-	out, outside
hemi-	half
hyper-	excessive, above
hypo-	deficient, under
in-	not
infra-	beneath, under
inter-	between
intra-	in, within, into
macro-	large
mal-	bad
meta-	beyond, change
micro-	small
neo-	new
pan-	all
para-	abnormal, beside, near
per-	through
peri-	surrounding
poly-	many, much
post-	after, behind
pre-	before, in front of
pro-	before, forward
pros-	before, forward
re-	back, again
retro-	behind, backward
sub-	under
supra-	above, upper
syn-, sym-	together, with
tachy-	fast
trans-	across, through
ultra-	beyond, excess
uni-	one

Suffix	Meaning	Suffix	Meaning
-cele	hernia	-cyte	cell
-dynia -algia	pain	-ectomy	to cut or remove
-emia	blood condition	-genesis	condition of producing, forming
-gram	record or image (such as an X-ray)	-graph	instrument for recording
-graphy	process of recording	-itis	inflammation
-logy	the study of	-lysis	breakdown, destruction, separation
-malacia	softening	-megaly	enlargement
-oma	tumor, mass, collection of fluid	-opsy	to view

Suffix	Meaning	Suffix	Meaning
-osis	abnormal condition	-pathy	disease condition
-penia	deficiency	-phobia	fear
-plasia	development, formation, growth	-plasty	surgical repair
-ptosis	drooping, falling, prolapse	-scopy -scopic	to look or observe
-stasis	controlling, stopping	-stomy	to make an opening or mouth
-therapy	treatment	-tomy	to cut into
-trophy	development, nourishment	-er	one who
-ia	condition	-ist	specialist
-ole	little, small	-ule	little, small
-um, -ium	structure, tissue	-us	structure, substance
-y	condition, process	-ac, -iac	pertaining to
-al	pertaining to	-ar	pertaining to
-ary	pertaining to	-ometer	an instrument measuring something
-genic	pertaining to, producing by or in	-ic, -ical	pertaining to
-oid	resembling, derived from	-ose, ous	pertaining to, full of
-ous	pertaining to	-tic	pertaining to

Before, we jump into root words, take a moment to ensure that you understand human body systems. There are several videos that review the components of the human body. If you have not had an opportunity to take anatomy and physiology in your coursework yet, or if you would like a quick review of the components of each body system, use the video collection link to access these videos before continuing with root word. Recall that one of the best ways to learn root words is to do so by body system so that words used in reference to these systems can be studied in groups.

Video Link Collection

Khan Academy Crash Course Anatomy Collection:

Digestive system: https://youtu.be/xtI1KcxR8Qs

Renal system, part 1: https://youtu.be/l128tW1H5a8

Urinary system, part 2: https://youtu.be/DlqyyyvTI3k

Respiratory system, part 1: https://youtu.be/bHZsvBdUC2I

Respiratory system, part 2: https://youtu.be/Cqt4LjHnMEA

Muscular system: https://youtu.be/5_6m0I1BUp4

Cardiovascular system, part 1: https://youtu.be/X9ZZ6tcxArI

Cardiovascular system, part 2: https://youtu.be/FLBMwcvOaEo

Circulatory system: https://youtu.be/9fxm85Fy4sQ

Skeletal system: https://youtu.be/RW46rQKWa-g

Nervous system: https://youtu.be/aP1KZzgR_dg

Integumentary system, part 1: https://youtu.be/Orumw-PyNjw

Integumentary system, part 2: https://youtu.be/EN-x-zXXVwQ

Lymphatic system: https://youtu.be/I7orwMgTQ5I
Endocrine system, part 1: https://youtu.be/eWHH9je2zG4
Endocrine system, part 2: https://youtu.be/SCV_m91mN-Q
Immune system: https://youtu.be/XZQDpzlENnk
Female reproductive system: https://youtu.be/RFDatCchpus
Male reproductive system: https://youtu.be/-XQcnO4iX_U

Now, let us look at specific words related to each body system. You can do this by reviewing the video collection provided in the preceding text or by following along in the tables provided in which words are grouped based on body system.

Medical terminology lesson collection:

https://www.youtube.com/playlist?list=PLRjNoiRtdFwUFUyEDPtXOzKH6KbQKF2Rc

The Study of Body Systems and Their Specialists

There are several fields of study that are unique to each body system as well as a specialist who is a health care provider trained in the management of diseases and conditions involving each body system. Like everything in health care, these fields of study and specialists have unique names. Review the following table. Note that the suffix, -ology refers to *the study of*, while -ologist refers to *a person who studies or specializes in something*.

Field of Study	Area of Study	Specialist	Area of Practice Specialty
Gynecology	the study of the female reproductive system	Gynecologist	a medical practitioner specializing in the diagnosis and treatment of the female reproductive system
Obstetrics	the study of pregnancy and childbirth	Obstetrician	a medical practitioner specializing in the diagnosis and treatment of pregnancy and childbirth
Gastroenterology	the study of the stomach and intestines	Gastroenterologist	a medical practitioner specializing in the diagnosis and treatment of the stomach and intestines
Cardiology	the study of the heart and vascular system	Cardiologist	a medical practitioner specializing in the diagnosis and treatment of heart
Endocrinology	the study of the endocrine system	Endocrinologist	a medical practitioner specializing in the diagnosis and treatment of endocrine glands and hormones
Pulmonology	the study of the respiratory system	Pulmonologist	a medical practitioner specializing in the diagnosis and treatment of the lungs
Orthopedics	the study of the musculoskeletal system	Orthopedist	a medical practitioner specializing in the diagnosis and treatment of congenital and functional abnormalities of muscle, joints, and bones
Dermatology	the study of the integumentary system	Dermatologist	a medical practitioner specializing in the diagnosis and treatment of the skin
Neurology	the study of the nervous system	Neurologist	a medical practitioner specializing in the diagnosis and treatment of the nervous system
Urology	the study of the renal system	Urologist	a medical practitioner specializing in the diagnosis and treatment of the renal system
Psychiatry	the study of mental, emotional, and abnormal disorders	Psychiatrist	a medical practitioner specializing in the diagnosis and treatment of mental disorders

Now that we have reviewed the fields involved in the study of the human body and the titles of those who specialize in these areas, let us now turn our attention to the actual body systems. As we review the system, note the special medical terminology used and its components.

Introduction to Digestive System Terminology

The oral cavity is the beginning of the digestive system

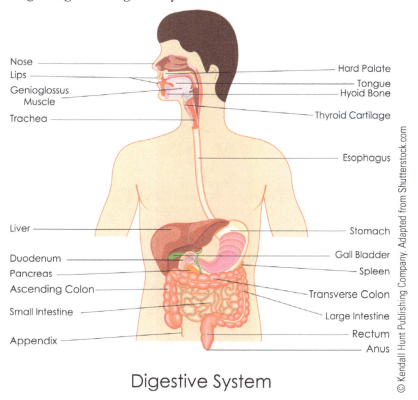

Digestive System

Oral cavity: where gastrointestinal tract begins

Tongue: extends across the floor of the oral cavity and muscles attach it to the lower jawbone

Pharynx: throat, the common passageway for food from the mouth and for air from the nose

Salivary Glands: parotid, sublingual, and submandibular glands

Esophagus: tube connecting the throat to stomach

Liver: large organ located in the right upper quadrant of the abdomen, secreted bile, stores sugar, iron, and vitamins

Stomach: muscular organ that receives food from the esophagus

Gallbladder: small sac under the liver, stores bile

Pancreas: organ behind the stomach, produces insulin and enzymes

Large intestine: extends from the end of the ileum to the anus

Small intestine: extends for 20 feet from the pyloric sphincter to the first part of the large intestine

Appendix: blind pouch hanging from the cecum in the right lower quadrant

Rectum: last section of the large intestine, connecting the end of the colon and the anus

Anus: terminal end or opening of the digestive tract to the outside of the body

Chapter 9 Introduction to Medical Terminology

Now let us look at the pathway that food takes through the body. Note in the following diagram how the digestive system is connected.

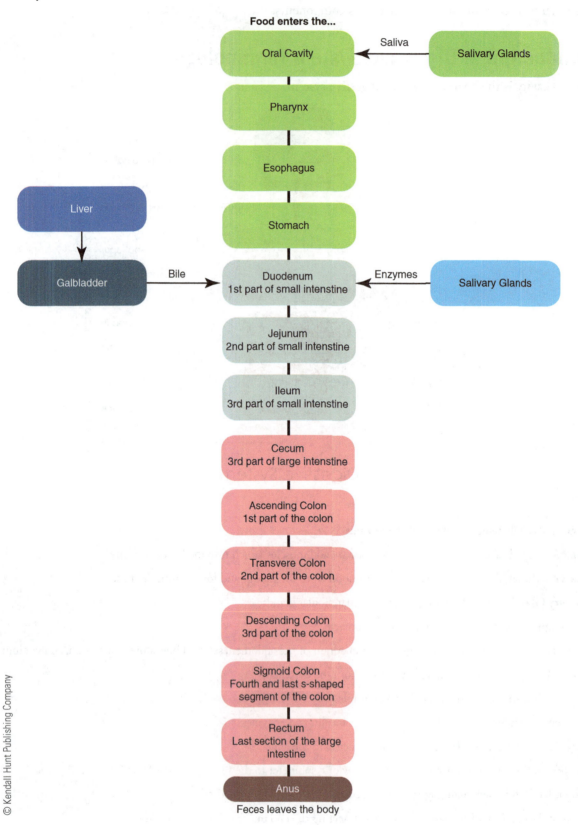

Knowing how this system works and functions, having used the above resources, let us take a look at the specific parts of the body using the *Combining Forms* and their meaning. Remember that the Combining Form is just a combination of the *Root* word and the *Combining Vowel*, put together.

Combining Form	Meaning	Combining Form	Meaning
an/o	anus	labi/o	lip
append/o	appendix	lapar/o	abdomen
bucc/o	cheek	lingu/o	tongue
cec/o	cecum	mandibul/o	lower jaw, mandible
celi/o	abdomen	odont/o	tooth
cheil/o	lip	or/o	mouth
cholecyst/o	gallbladder	palat/o	palate
choledoch/o	common bile duct	pancreat/o	pancreas
col/o	colon	peritone/o	peritoneum
dent/i/o	teeth	p	throat
duoden/o	duodenum	proct/o	anus and rectum
enter/o	intestine, usually small intestine	pylor/o	pyloric sphincter
esophag/o	esophagus	rect/o	rectum
faci/o	face	sailaden/o	salivary gland
gastr/o	stomach	sigmoid/o	sigmoid colon
gingiv/o	gums	stomat/o	mouth
gloss/o	tongue	uvul/o	uvula
hepat/o	liver	lingu/o	tongue
ile/o	ileum	jejun/o	jejunum

Here are a few suffixes that are generally used with digestive system combining forms.

Suffix	Meaning		
-ase	enzyme	-plasty	surgical repair
-chezia	defecation, elimination	-ptysis	spitting
-iasis	abnormal condition	-rrhage/rrhagia	bursting forth
-prandial	meal	-rrhaphy	suture
-ectasis	dilation	-rrhea	flow, discharge
-ectasia	widening	-spasm	involuntary contraction of muscle
-emesis	vomiting	-stasis	stopping, controlling
-pepsia	digestion	-stenosis	narrowing, tightening
-phagia	eating, swallowing	-tresia	opening

Common Body Fluid and Substance Combining Forms

Combining Form	Meaning	Combining Form	Meaning
amyl/o	starch	lip/o	fat, lipid
bil/i	gall, bile	lith/o	stone
bilirubin/o	bilirubin	prote/o	protein
chol/e	gall, bile	py/o	pus
chlorhydr/o	hydrochloric acid	sial/o	saliva, salivary
gly/o, gluc/o	sugar	steat/o	fat
glycogen/o		glycogen, animal starch	

When learning medical words, it is also helpful to understand the different kinds of laboratory tests and clinical procedures you may encounter in your studies. Here are a few laboratory tests and clinical procedures described for you to increase your foundational knowledge.

Test/Procedure	Definition
Hemoccult or Guiac Test	test to detect occult blood in feces
Cholangiography	x-ray examination of the biliary system performed after injection of contrast into the bile ducts
Computed Tomography (CT)	a series of x-ray images taken in multiple views and then placed in a 4D model
Abdominal Ultrasonography	sound waves beamed into the abdomen to produce an image of the abdominal cavity
Endoscopic Ultrasonography	use of an endoscope combined with an ultrasound to examine organs in the GI tract
Magnetic Resonance Imaging (MRI)	magnetic waves that produce images of organs and tissues in all three planes of the body
Gastrointestinal Endoscopy	visual examination of the gastrointestinal tract using an endoscope
Laparoscopy	visual examination of the abdomen with a laparoscope inserted through small incisions in the abdomen

Introduction to Urinary System Terminology

Combining Form	Meaning	Combining Form	Meaning
cali/o, calic/o	calys; cup-shaped	pyle/o	renal pelvis
cyst/o	urinary bladder	ren/o	kidney
glomerul/o	glomerulus	trigon/o	trigone (a region of the bladder)
meat/o	meatus	ureter/o	ureter
nephr/o	kidney	urethr/o	urethra
vesic/o		urinary bladder	

Here are a few laboratory tests and clinical procedures described for you to increase your foundational knowledge of the urinary system.

Test/Procedure	Definition
Urinalysis	A laboratory test that examines the urine to identify abnormal components which help inform health, infection, or potential disease processes.
CT Urography	X-ray images using the CT machine which combines and forms a 4D cross-sectional view.

Test/Procedure	Definition
KUB (kidney ureter and bladder)	A specific x-ray of the kidneys, ureters, and the bladder.
RP Retrograde pyelogram	An x-ray image that shows the renal structures which is done by injecting a contrast material into the system using a urinary catheter.
Cystoscopy	Using a small tube with a camera on the end of it to visualize the ureters and bladder.
Dialysis	A procedure that involves exchanging a person's blood through a filter device and returning it to the body to separate and remove nitrous waste. This process is an artificial way of performing kidney waste elimination functions.
Lithotripsy	A procedure in which renal stones are crushed or pulverized.
Urinary Catheterization	Inserting a small flexible tube through the urethra and into the bladder for the purpose of collecting urine.

Introduction to Cardiovascular System Terminology

Let us take a moment to review the function of blood vessels and the circulatory process of the blood through the human body.

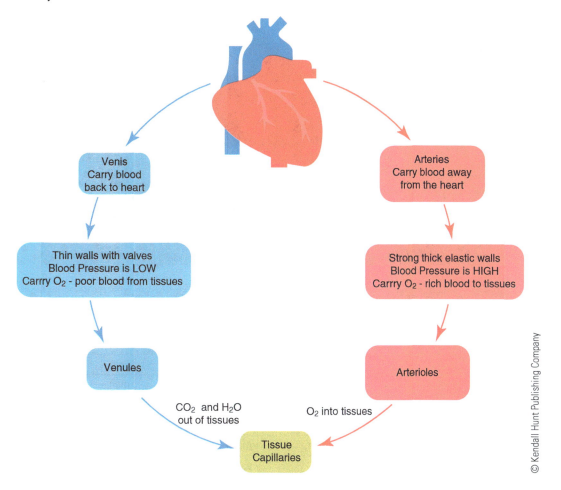

In the preceding and following diagrams, note that the red arrows refer to oxygenated blood and the blue arrows refer to blood that is oxygen poor. Notice the flow of the blood from the lungs through the heart. Here we see delivery of oxygenated blood to organs and tissues and then oxygen poor blood returning to the heart and lungs to begin the process all over again. This process is referred to as *the cardiopulmonary process* because it involves this constant cycle. Because of this, the cardiovascular system has many root words and combining forms that are specific to the heart, the blood vessel, the chest cavity, as well as colors, locations, and effects of the system such as the heart rhythm and pulse.

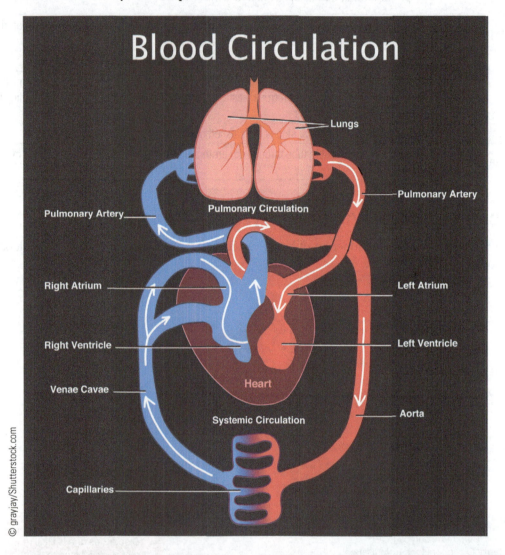

© grayjay/Shutterstock.com

Combining Form	Meaning	Combining Form	Meaning
angi/o	vessel	ox/o	oxygen
aort/o	aorta	pericardi/o	pericardium
arter/o, arteri/o	artery	phleb/o	vein
ather/o	yellowish plaque, fatty substance	rrhythm/o	rhythm
atri/o	atrium, upper heart chamber	sphygm/o	pulse
brachi/o	arm	steth/o	chest
cardi/o	heart	thromb/o	clot
cholesterol/o	cholesterol	valvul/o,	valve
coron/o	heart	valv/o	valve
cyan/o	blue	vascul/o	vessel
myx/o	mucus	ven/o, ven/i	vein
vas/o	vessel	ventricul/o	ventricle, lower heart chamber

Let us take a moment now and see if we can figure out the meaning of a piece of equipment used in health care. What is a sphygmomanometer? First break the word into components like this: sphygm/o—manometer. Let me start by determining what a manometer is. A *manometer* is a noun because it is an object. Used in many fields, a manometer is an instrument that measures the pressure of fluid. Now, using the preceding combining form table, can you determine what kind of fluid pressure we would be measuring in the cardiovascular system? *Sphygm/o* refers to your pulse. Therefore, when we put these two ideas together, we come up with a measurement of our blood pulse pressure. In health care, this is referred to simply as *blood pressure* and the piece of equipment that we use to take your blood pressure is referred to as a sphygmomanometer. Learning how to break words apart to understand their individual component meaning allows us to quickly understand words we may have never seen before.

How about the word, pericarditis? Once again, break the word into its components, like this: *peri-card-itis*. Do you remember our rules from the beginning of the chapter? Let us have a quick review: (1) *Read*, (2) *Drop*, and (3) *Keep*. *Read* the meaning of the medical word from the suffix back to the beginning of the word. Second, *drop* the combining vowel (in most cases it is an "o" before a suffix that begins with a vowel. Third, *keep* the combining vowel between two roots in any word. So let us go back to our word, *pericarditis*. Start at the end with *itis*. Recall that this suffix means "inflammation of." Do we have a combining vowel? In this instance we do not. We can clearly see that the combining form is *cardi*, meaning heart. When we put the root and suffix together it means: inflammation of the heart. But wait! We still have that prefix to add to the word. Recall that a prefix can change the meaning of the word, so we do not ever want to forget to add it back in. In this example, our prefix is *peri*. If we go back to our main prefix table we see that *peri* means, surrounding. When we add the prefix, it does change the meaning. By adding *peri* to *carditis* we no longer mean that the heart is inflamed, rather, it is the area around the outside of the heart that is inflamed. In fact, one of the areas surrounding the heart is called the *pericardium*! The pericardium is the membrane that encapsulates the heart. Think of it like a big sack that contains the heart muscle itself. See the difference? The word pericarditis is a great example of why you not only have to take science classes, like anatomy and physiology, but you have to retain the information. In understanding medical terminology, you need more than a simple ability to break the word down; you need foundational sciences like anatomy that will help you determine the exact meaning. Every single class that you take as a prerequisite FOR a nursing program is extremely valuable to your success IN a nursing program. For more information on pericarditis you can read the information provided by the American Heart Association: https://www.heart.org/en/health-topics/pericarditis/what-is-pericarditis.

Test/Procedure	Definition
Cardiac biomarkers	A series of blood tests that help identify if a person is undergoing a heart attack
Angiography	An x-ray image that allows a clinician to see the vessels of the heart after injecting a contrast material into the circulatory system
Doppler ultrasound	Sound waves that measure blood flow within blood vessels
Echo	High frequency sound waves that produce an image of the inside of the heart
Cardiac catheterization	A small tube that is inserted in a large vein or artery and is guided into the heart for intervention
Electrocardiography (EKG)	This procedure involves using small stickers and cables on the outside of the body to detect the electrical activity of the heart. This electrical activity pattern forms your heartbeat and is captured on either a computer screen or can be printed out on a piece of paper.
Stress test	This is a physical exertion test, usually conducted on a treadmill that helps clinicians understand a person's tolerance to increasing levels of physical activity while being monitored.

Specific Terminology Related to the Blood

Take a moment to review the cellular level of the blood in the diagram provided. Many of the words we use in reference to a test or lab result, a patient's condition, or a patient's symptoms have to do with blood results. Provided for you is a table of combining forms specifically used with lab work and their associated suffixes.

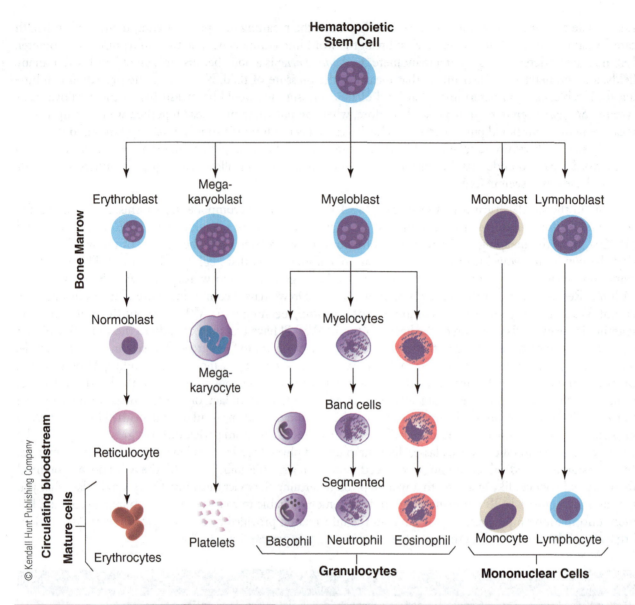

Combining Form	Meaning	Combining Form	Meaning
bas/o	base	leuk/o	white
chrom/o	color	mon/o	one, single
coagul/o	clotting	morph/o	shape, form
cyt/o/e	cell	myel/o	bone marrow
eosin/o	red, dawn, rosy	neutr/o	neutral
erythr/o	red	nucle/o	nucleus
granul/o	granules	phag/o	eat, swallow
hem/o	blood	poikil/o	varied, irregular
hemat/o	blood	sider/o	iron
hemoglobin/o	hemoglobin	spher/o	globe, round
is/o	same, equal	thromb/o	clot
kary/o		nucleus	

Suffix	Meaning	Suffix	Meaning
-apheresis	removal, carrying away	-oid	derived or originating from
-blast	immature or embryonic cell	-osis	abnormal condition
-cytosis	abnormal condition of cell	-penia	deficiency
-emia	blood condition	-phage	eat, swallow
-gen	giving rise to; producing	-philia	attraction for
-globin	protein	-phoresis	carrying, transmission
-lytic	pertaining to destruction	-stasis	stop, control

Learning words that are able to help us understand the cellular level, especially when we are discussing a patient's blood is quite helpful. As nurses you will not only be responsible for obtaining blood and fluid samples correctly, you will also be required to interpret laboratory results, critically think through the results applying their meaning to the patient's condition, and appropriately notify care providers for further treatment orders if necessary. Let us look at a few laboratory terms that refer to blood tests to see if we can determine what is being analyzed or what condition a patient may have as it pertains to his or her blood. The word *hemoglobin* is a component of a red blood cell. Let us discover what it is by breaking down the word. The suffix in this word is represented by *globin* and refers to protein; *hem/o* represents the combining form meaning blood. Together, *hemoglobin* refers to a component of the red blood cell that stores proteins. Let us try another. What does the word *thrombocytopenia* refer to? The suffix is *penia* and means deficiency. There are two combining forms in this word. The first, *thromb/o* refers to a clot in the blood and the second *cyt/o* means cell. Together thrombocytopenia means a deficiency of the blood cell's clotting ability or someone whose blood cells do not clot properly. Finally, let us determine what kind of blood cell the following word represents. Take a moment to break apart the word *leukocyte*. In this word we have two combining forms: *leuk/o* meaning white and *cyte* meaning cell. The word *leukocyte* refers to white blood cells. White blood cells are named for their appearance when observed under a microscope. These cells protect you against illness and disease.

Introduction to Respiratory System Terms

Let us take a moment to review the function of the lungs in the human body. In the following respiratory section, we will clearly learn not only combining forms for parts of the respiratory system such as the lungs, diaphragm, and trachea but we will also be reviewing colors, gases, and sound components as well.

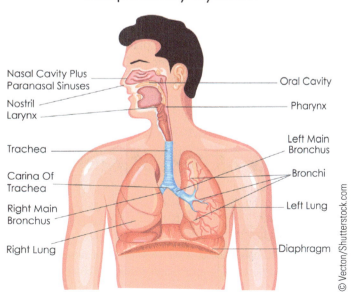

Combining Form	Meaning	Combining Form	Meaning
adenoid/o	adenoids	vertig/o	dizziness
alveol/o	alveolus, air sac	pector/o	chest
bronch/o, bronchi/o	bronchial tube, bronchus	pharyng/o	pharynx, throat
bronchiol/o	bronchiole, small bronchus	phon/o	voice
capn/o	carbon dioxide	phren/o	diaphragm
coni/o	dust	pleur/o	pleura
cyan/o	blue	pneum/o, pneumon/o, pulm/o	air, lung
epiglott/o	epiglottis	rhin/o	nose
laryng/o	larynx, voice box	sinus/o	sinus, cavity
lob/o	lobe of the lung	spir/o	breathing
mediastin/o	mediastinum	tel/o	complete
nas/o	nose	thorac/o	chest
orth/o	straight, upright	tonsill/o	tonsils
pnea	breath, respiration	trache/o	trachea, wind pipe

Suffix	Meaning
-ema	condition
-osmia	smell
-pnea	breathing
-ptysis	spitting
-sphyxia	pulse
-thorax	pleural cavity, chest
-ia	disease or pathologic condition

Given the word prefix/suffix and combining forms in the preceding tables, if a patient were to complain of orthopnea, what would the complaint involve? The combining forms of *orth/o* meaning upright and *pnea*, meaning breath or respiration, are placed together in this term. *Orthopnea* is the term associated with a sensation of breathlessness when someone is reclined; thus, the condition improves when the person stands or sits upright. Let us try another word. What happens when a patient complains of *dyspnea*? The combining form is *pnea* once again meaning breath or respiration and it is joined by the prefix *dys*, meaning bad, painful, and abnormal. In this instance, the patient is complaining of difficult or painful breathing. Finally, let us try the word *laryngitis*. The suffix is *itis*, meaning inflammation; *laryng/o* is the combining form referring to the anatomical structure, the larynx. The combining vowel is dropped. The word *laryngitis* means inflammation of the larynx which we often associate with "losing your voice."

Test/Procedure	Definition
Chest x-ray (CXR) anterior posterior and lateral (A/P & LAT)	Radiographic image of the chest cavity which includes the lungs and the directions to the technician on how to take the x-ray include taking the film anterior-posterior to obtain the view of the chest from the front to the back of the chest as well as from the side of the patient, shoulder to shoulder to ensure all fields of the lungs are observed.
Bronchoscopy	A small fiber-optic endoscope with a camera that allows a clinician to visualize the bronchial passage of the lungs.

Test/Procedure	Definition
Pulmonary function tests (PFTs)	These include a group of tests that allow clinicians to measure the ventilation ability of the lungs. It includes lung volume, airway function, and lung capacity (exchanging O_2 and CO_2).
Thoracentesis	A surgical procedure that removes fluid from the pleural space.
Tracheostomy	A surgical creation of a small hole or opening directly into the trachea through the front of the neck.

Introduction to Nervous System Terms

The nervous system is one of the most complex human body systems. Terminology for the nervous system can be extensive and include a number of patient signs and symptoms related to abnormal conditions experienced by people with alterations in this system.

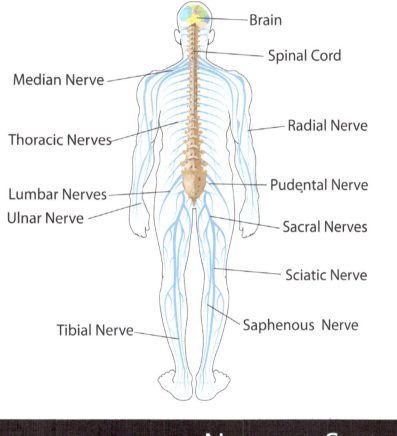

© snapgalleria/Shutterstock.com

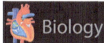

Combining Form	Meaning	Suffix	Meaning
alges/o, algesia	sensitivity to pain	-algia	pain
caus/o	burning	-lepsy	seizure
comat/o	deep sleep (coma)	-paresis	weakness
esthesi/o	feeling, nervous sensation	-esthesia	feeling, nervous sensation
kines/o, kinesi/o, kinesis	movement	-kinesia, kinetic	movement

(*continued*)

Chapter 9 Introduction to Medical Terminology

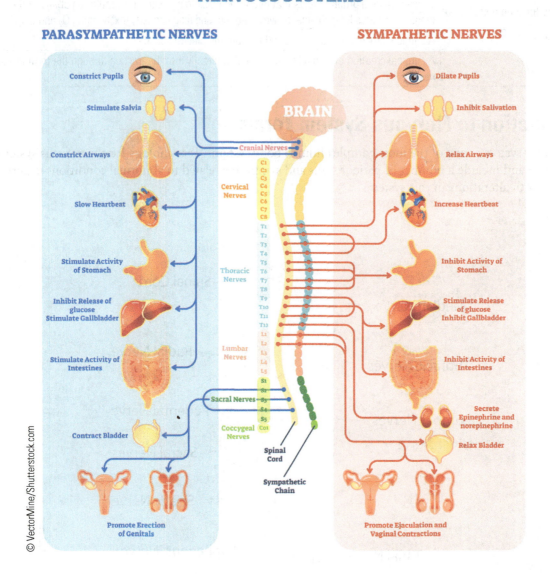

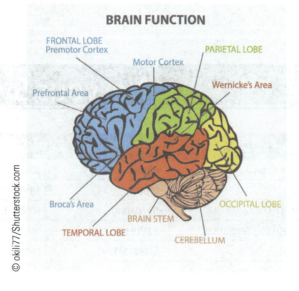

Combining Form	Meaning	Suffix	Meaning
lex/o	word, phrase	-phasia	speech
syncop/o	to cut off, cut short	-plegia	paralysis
tax/o	order, coordination	-praxia	action
mening/i/o	membrane	-sthenia	strength
neur/o	nerve	-malacia	softening
crani/o	skull	-gram	to record or an image
cephal/a/o	head	-oma	tumor, mass, collection of fluid
electr/o	electricity	-phagia	eating or swallowing

Breaking down complex nervous system words should not be a challenge if you remember to use the rule! Read, Drop, Keep.

Let us practice with a few examples of common words you will see referring to the nervous system in health care settings. Craniotomy: *otomy* is the suffix and means to cut into; *crani/o* is the combining form and refers to the skull. The word craniotomy means to surgically cut into the skull. Cephalahematoma: *oma* is the suffix and in this instance means a collection of fluid; there are actually two different combining forms in this word: *cephal/a*, which means head and *hem/a*, which means blood. Do not let this fool you even though it seems complex. The word *cephalahematoma* refers to a collection of blood between the scalp and the skull. This is another instance when determining the exact meaning of the medical term requires a solid foundation in anatomy and physiology (A&P). Within having had the course A&P one might only be able to determine that a cephalahematoma is a collection of blood on the head. This is close but does not capture the exact intension of the word. Neuritis: *itis* is the suffix; *neur/o* is the combining form and means nerve. The word *neuritis* means inflammation of a nerve. Meningitis: *itis* is the suffix; *mening/o* is the combining form and refers to the meninges which are three membranes that line the skull and spine that encapsulate the brain and spinal cord. If you have never taken the course A&P would you know what is inflamed in this word? The word *meningitis* means inflammation of the meninges. Electroencephalogram (EEG): *gram* is the suffix and means to record; there are two combining forms in this word: *electr/o* meaning electric and *cephal/o* meaning head; the prefix is *en* meaning, in or within. The word *electroencephalogram* means to record the electrical signals within the head. This is a test that tracks and records brain wave patterns or brain function. Neuromalacia: *malacia* is the suffix and means softening; *neur/o* is the combining form and means nerve. The word *neuromalacia* literally means a softening of the nerve or nerve tissue which is often pathologic (diseased) in nature.

Test/Procedure	Definition
EEG electroencephalography	Recording the electrical activity of the brain
LP lumbar puncture	Removing a small sample of CSF, with a needle, between two vertebrae, for analysis
CSF cerebrospinal analysis	Lab test in which a sample of CSF is examined for abnormalities

Introduction to Musculoskeletal System Terminology

Musculoskeletal system refers to both the bones of the human body as well as the numerous muscles that cover and give shape to the body. This is an important system because it is what allows a person to move and to have strength with movement. The musculoskeletal system also protects vital organs and produces blood cells. Your understanding of the components, conditions, and symptoms associated with this system are integral to your role. Let us begin with a review of the following diagrams showing in the first the skeletal structure followed by the placement of muscle over the skeletal frame.

Chapter 9 Introduction to Medical Terminology

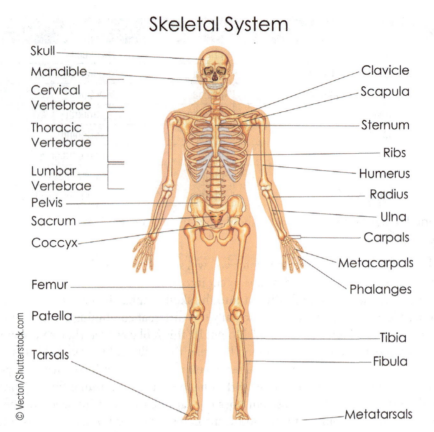

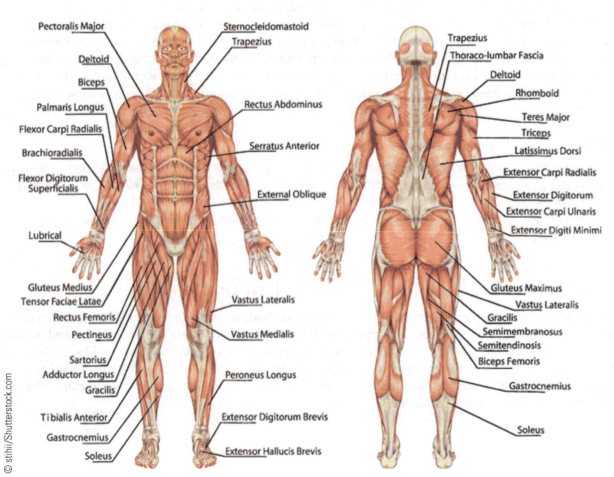

There are numerous words associated with the musculoskeletal system largely in part to the sheer number of muscles and bones in the human body. Imagine that as a nurse, you will have to document and discuss orthopedic (refers to the correction of deformities in the muscle and bone) complaints and conditions with patients and their families. You will need to provide education regarding these conditions and understand the kind of surgeries and procedures that they will have completed in the operating room or doctor's office. Let us begin by looking at common combining forms in regarding the musculoskeletal system.

Combining Form	Meaning	Combining Form	Meaning
disk/o	disk or disc	rachi/o	spine
fasci/o	fascia, band	radi/o	radius
femor/o	femur	rhabd/o	striated muscle
fibul/o	fibula	sacr/o	sacrum
humer/o	humerus	scapula/o	scapula
ili/o	ilium	scoli/o	crooked, twisted
ischi/o	ischium	stern/o	sternum
kinesi/o, kinet/o	movement	synovi/o	synovial fluid or joint
kyph/o	humpback	tars/o	tarsal bone
dactyl/o	finger or digit	ten/o	tendon
lamin/o	lamina	tend/o	tendon
lord/o	curved, bent	tendin/o	tendon
lumb/o	lumbar region, lower back	thorac/o	thorax or chest
mandibul/o	mandible	ton/o	tone or tension
maxilla/o	maxilla	uln/o	ulna
minisc/o	meniscus	vertebr/o	vertebra
my/o	muscle	spondyl/o	vertebra
myel/o	bone marrow, spinal cord	myos/o	muscle
oste/o	bone	muscul/o	muscle
patell/o	patella	phalang/o	
pelv/i/o	pelvis, pelvic cavity	pub/o	

There are also several prefixes and suffixes common to the musculoskeletal system.

Prefix	Meaning
inter-	between
intra-	within
supra-	above
sub-	below, beneath
sym-, syn-	together, with

Suffix	Meaning
-algia	pain
-asthenia	weakness
-centesis	puncture to remove or aspirate what's within
-clasia, -clasis, -clast	to break
-desis	surgical fixation, binding

(*continued*)

Suffix	Meaning
-ectomy	surgical removal
-it is	inflammation of
-osis	abnormal condition
-physis	growth
-plasty	surgical repair, reconstruction of
-porosis	pore or passage
-rrhaphy	suture
-schisis	to split
-trophy	development, nourishment

Let us take a moment to practice breaking down a few musculoskeletal words commonly found in this field. In breaking down the word scoliosis, we note that the suffix is *osis* which means an abnormal condition. The combining form in this example is *scoli/o* which refers to crooked or twisted. In the field of orthopedics, *scoliosis* refers to an abnormal condition of the spine in which it is twisted or crooked. What then would you think the word *lordosis* means? Still referring to the spine, what do we find when we break the word down into its components? The suffix again is *osis*, which means abnormal condition. The combining form is *lord/o* which means curved or bent. The word *lordosis* literally means an abnormal condition in which the spine is curved or bent. In our third example of the description of the spine let us look at the word *kyphosis*. Again, the suffix is *osis* meaning an abnormal condition. The combining form is *kyph/o* which translates to humpback. The word *kyphosis* means an abnormal condition of the spine in which a humpback pattern appears. See the illustrations below to understand a visual representation of the difference between kyphosis, scoliosis, and lordosis.

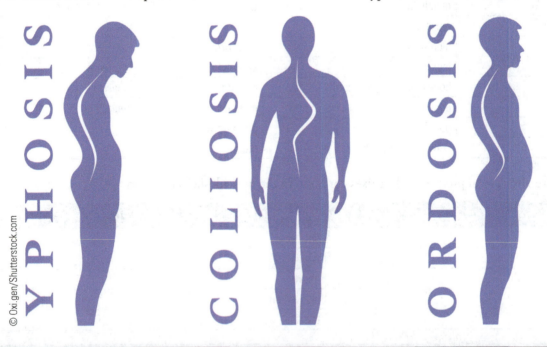

Tests/Procedures	Meaning
Arthrography	the use of a contrast material to identify abnormalities on x-ray
Arthroscopy	a surgical procedure in which a small camera scope is inserted into the interior of a joint
Bone scan	an image obtained by using a small amount of a radioactive material that highlights the bone so that disorders can be identified
Bone densitometry	an x-ray technique that determines the density of a person's bone useful in diagnosing bone conditions

Introduction to Female and Male Reproductive System Terminology

The reproductive system of the human body is divided into two distinct systems: the female reproductive system and the male reproductive system. Let us first review the following diagrams of each system. Because each system is distinct, terminology related to each system is unique and reflects not only the anatomy but the body fluid and reproductive process.

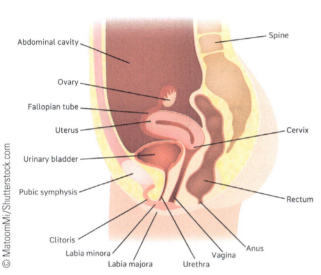

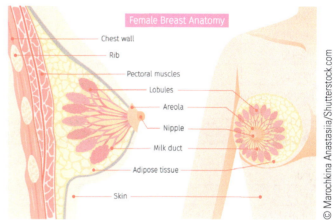

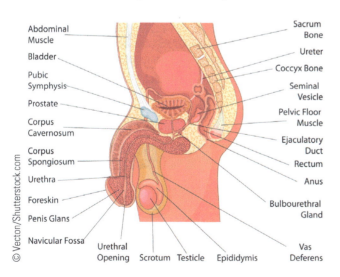

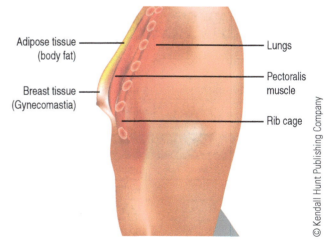

Female Combining Form	Meaning	Female Combining Form	Meaning
amni/o	amnion	my/o	muscle
cervic/o	cervix, neck	nat/i	birth
chori/o, chorion/o	chorion	obstetr/o	pregnancy
colp/o	vagina	o/o	egg
culd/o	cul-de-sac	oophor/o	ovary
episi/o	vulva	ov/o	egg
galact/o	milk	ovari/o	ovary
gynec/o	woman, female	ovul/o	egg
hyster/o	uterus	perine/o	perineum
lact/o	milk	phoro/o	to bear
mamm/o	breast	salping/o	fallopian tube
mast/o	breast	uter/o	uterus
men/o	menses, menstruation	vagin/o	vagina
metro/o, metri/o	uterus	vulv/o	vulva

Female Prefix	Meaning	Female Suffix	Meaning
dys-	painful	-arche	beginning
endo-	within	-cyesis	pregnancy
in-	In	-gravida	pregnant
intra-	within	-parous	bearing, bringing forth
multi-	many	-rrhea	flow or discharge
nulli-	no, not, none	-salpinx	fallopian tube
pre-	before	-tocia	labor, birth
primi-	first	-version	act of turning
retro-	backward		

Male Combining Form	Meaning	Male Combining Form	Meaning
andr/o	male	prostat/o	prostate gland
balan/o	glans penis	sperm/o, sperat/o	sperm
orchid/o, orchi/o, orch/o	testis, testicle	vas/o	vessel, duct
epididym/o	epididymis	test/o	testis, testicle

Male Prefix	Meaning
dys-	painful, abnormal, difficult, labored
endo-	within
epi-	on, upon, over
eu-	normal or good
hyper-	above, excessive
hypo-	below, incomplete, deficient
intra-	within
meta-	after, beyond, change
trans-	through, across, beyond
oligo-	a few or scant amount

Male Suffix	Meaning	Male Suffix	Meaning
-cele	hernia or protrusion	-scopy	to look or observe
-centesis	surgical procedure to aspirate fluid	-spasm	sudden, involuntary muscle contraction
-ectasis	stretching out, dilation, expansion	-stenosis	constriction or narrowing
-graphy	process of recording	-stomy	a created opening
-ism	state of	-scope	an instrument for inspecting or viewing
-meter	instrument used to measure	-scopic	to look or observe
-metry	measurement	-rrhagia	rapid flow of blood
-pexy	surgical fixation, suspension	-in	stuff

Reproductive Tests/Procedures	Definition
Male: Transrectal Ultrasound	Use of sound waves to diagnose prostate cancer, across the rectum view
Male: PSA (prostate-specific antigen)	A laboratory test that measures a specific protein exclusively produced by prostate cells
Male: DRE (digital rectal examination)	A digital procedure by a clinician to feel the size and shape of the prostate gland through the rectal wall
Female: Pap Test	Routine lab test screening for cervical cancer involving the staining of cervical cells removed from the vagina and cervix to be examined under a microscope
Female: Pregnancy Test	A lab test via a blood sample or urine sample that detects the presence of hCG
Female: Mammography	Routine screening: X-ray image of breast tissue
Female: Colposcopy	A special instrument that is used to closely examine the cervix, vagina, and vulva for abnormalities
Female: Amniocentesis	Laboratory test involving the microscopic puncturing of the amniotic sac of a pregnant woman. The amniotic fluid withdrawn is analyzed for abnormality and treatment

Let us practice breaking down both female and male reproductive terminology. Remember to use the rule: *Read, Drop, Keep*. Anorchism: *ism* is the suffix and means the state of; *orchi/o* is the combining form and means testis; *an/o* means without. The word *anorchism* means: the state of absence of testis. Epididymitis: *itis* is the suffix and means inflammation; *epididym/o* is the combining form and refers to a body part in the male reproductive system called the *epididymis*. The word *epididymitis* means inflammation of the epididymis. Prostatocystitis: *itis* is the suffix and means inflammation; *prostate/o* is the combining form and refers to a body part in the male reproductive system called the *prostate gland*; *cyst/o* means urinary bladder. The word *prostatocystitis* means inflammation of the prostate gland and the urinary bladder. Prostatorrhea: *rrhea* is the suffix and means flow or discharge; *prostat/o* is the combining form and refers to a part in the male reproductive system called the *prostate gland*. The word prostatorrhea means discharge from the prostate gland. Spermatolysis: *lysis* is the suffix and means dissolution or destruction; *spermat/o* is the combining form and refers to *sperm*. The word *spermatolysis* means destruction of sperm. Oligospermia: *olig/o* is the suffix and means a few or scant amount; *sperm/o* is the combining form and refers to sperm. The word *oligospermia* means having a scant amount of sperm. Amenorrhea: *rrhea* is the suffix and means discharge or flow; *men/o* is the combining form and refers to female menses; the prefix *a* means without. The word *amenorrhea* means the absence of menses. Cervicitis: *itis* is the suffix and means inflammation; *cervic/o* is the combining form and refers to the female reproductive body part called the *cervix*. In this instance we drop the combining vowel. The word *cervicitis* means inflammation of the cervix. Dysmenorrhea: *rrhea* is the suffix and means discharge or flow; *men/o* is the combining form and refers to female menses; the prefix *dys* means painful. The word *dysmenorrhea* means painful menstruation.

Introduction to Integumentary System Terminology

The integumentary system refers to more than just the human skin layer. As you will note in the diagram it is a full interdependent protective system. The skin actually is comprised of three layers: the epidermis (outer layer through which hair grows) and dermis (inner layer) and a subcutaneous layer known as the hypodermis, as noted in the diagram. The dermis contains glands that secrete various byproducts like ear wax, sweat, and oil. This body system contains medical terminology that relates to these structures, including symptoms and its assessment such as color, elasticity, and texture. Associated conditions of the integument are also included in this section which refers to any pathology or disease process such as a cancer or burn.

THE STRUCTURE OF THE SKIN

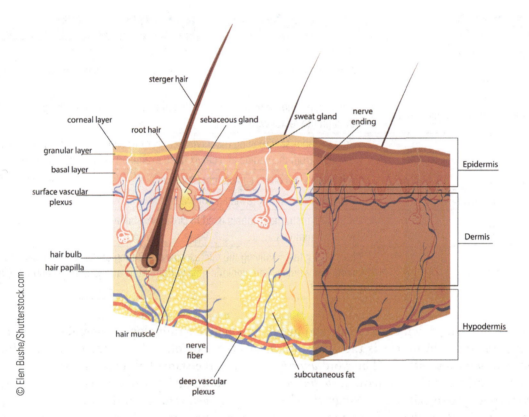

© Elen Bushe/Shutterstock.com

Let us take a closer look at common combining forms: prefixes and suffixes used with the integumentary system.

Combining Form	Meaning
cut/a/o-	skin
derm/a/o- dermat/o	skin
lip/o	fat
melan/o	black
cyan/o	blue
xanth/o	yellow
onych/i/o	nail
scler/o	hard/tough
sudor/o	sweat
carcin/o	cancer

Prefix	Meaning	Suffix	Meaning
pachy-	thick	-itis	inflammation of
super-	above, in addition, over	-oma	tumor, mass, collection of fluid
sub-	under, beneath	-osis	condition or disease
supra-	above, on the upper side	-ogen	precursor
pseudo-	false, fake	-ific	creating or causing
epi-	on, up, against, high	-us	structure or thing
phyto	of plant origin		

Take a moment to practice a few commonly used integumentary system words in nursing and health care. Remember, many of the words will describe the skin or the location of skin, a problem with the skin such as a lump or a condition of the skin such as a burn or pathologic process. Subcutaneous: *ous* is the suffix and means structure or thing; *cut/a* is the combining form and means skin; *sub* is the prefix and refers to beneath or under. The word *subcutaneous* means below the structure of the skin or below the skin layer. Dermatology: *logy* is the suffix and means the study of; *dermat/o* is the combining form meaning skin. The word *dermatology* refers to the study of skin. Lipoma: *oma* is the suffix and means tumor or mass; *lip/o* is the combining form and means fat. The word *lipoma* refers to a tumor or mass in the skin made of fat. Melanocyte: *cyt/e* is the combining form and means cell; *melan/o* is also a combining form which refers to the color black. Together the word *melanocyte* means a cell that appears black.

Onchyectomy: *ectomy* is the suffix which means to remove; *onchy/o* is the combining form and refers to your finger or toenail. In this instance we drop the combining vowel. The word *onchyectomy* means to remove a (toe or finger) nail. Pachyderma: The combining form is *derm/a* and means skin; the prefix in the word is *pachy* which means thick. The word *pachyderma* refers to abnormal thickening of the skin. Sudorific: *ific* is the suffix and means creating or causing; *sudor/o* is the combining form and refers to sweat. In this case we drop the combining vowel. The word *sudorific* refers to something that causes or creates sweat. Dermatophytosis: *osis* is the suffix and refers to a condition or disease; *dermat/o* is the combining form meaning skin; *phyto* is the prefix which literally means of plant origin. This is another example of why it is important to retain scientific course information as this literal translation may leave you scratching your head. The word does not mean a skin disease caused by a plant, but it is close. *Dermatophytosis* refers to a fungal infection of the skin.

Putting Medical Terminology in Context

The ability to take what you have learned and apply it in a real patient situation is the ultimate goal of learning medical terminology. As nurses we are responsible for writing the correct medical term for a procedure on consent forms; being able to read and understand the contents of a medical note; as well as, competently document our own assessment findings using the standardized language found in all clinical settings. While this may seem like a daunting task, take a moment to review the medical note below, which has been provided to help your ability to synthesize the content in this chapter. Complete the following learning activities to ensure comprehension.

Practice Example 1

Read the following paragraph out loud. Break down the highlighted words using the rules discussed in this chapter: Read, Drop, Keep. Which body system is the paragraph referring to? Define each word that is highlighted and then rewrite the paragraph so that you are replacing the medical words with their meaning. Can you rephrase the medical paragraph into a passage that could easily be understood by someone with a low health literacy level? What is the patient in the emergency room for? What is her medical history? Why is she being admitted? What tests has she had done. Can you interpret the abbreviations used in the paragraph?

A 72 year-old female, with NKA, who complains of **dyspnea** and **vertigo** on admission. The patient has a history of **carcinoma**, which was successfully removed in 2019, and a reoccurring **lipoma** to her left leg. Additionally, her medical history reveals persistent **neuritis** to her right foot x 15 years as well as **pyelonephritis** in 2018 which resolved with antibiotics. On room air, the patient's oxygen saturation is 78%. She reports falling at home with the vertiginous episode and sustaining a **hematoma** to her left shoulder and forehead. Her vital signs reveal persistent **bradypnea** and an irregular heartbeat. She currently c/o being unable to "catch her breath." The patient has undergone an **EKG**, which revealed intermittent atrial fibrillation, and is scheduled for a portable **CXR, A/P & LAT** stat. The patient will be seen by the on-call **pulmonologist, cardiologist** and **neurologist** before being transferred to the medical floor for observation. The patient had been seen by respiratory therapy and has been placed on oxygen. She has additionally been instructed to use her incentive **spirometer** while awake. The patient will be maintained at bedrest and will be closely monitored.

Ans Key:

Dyspnea	Bad or difficult breathing
Vertigo	Dizziness
Carcinoma	Cancer tumor or mass
Lipoma	Fat tumor or mass
Neuritis	Inflammation of a nerve
Pyelonephritis	Inflammation of renal pelvis and kidneys
Hematoma	Collection of blood
Bradypnea	Slow breathing
EKG	Electrocardiogram
CXR, A/P & LAT	Chest x-ray taken using views anterior/posterior and lateral
Pulmonologist	A medical practitioner specializing in the diagnosis and treatment of the lungs
Cardiologist	A medical practitioner specializing in the diagnosis and treatment of heart
Neurologist	A medical practitioner specializing in the diagnosis and treatment of the nervous system
Spirometer	Instrument used to measure breathing

Practice Example 2

Write the meaning of the prefix or suffix provided below:

-schisis	
-ectomy	
pachy-	
sub-	

-osis	
-rrhea	
-sphyxia	
-ema	
a-	
micro-	
brady-	

Ans Key:

-Schisis	to split
-Ectomy	surgical removal
Pachy-	thick
Sub-	below or beneath
-Osis	condition or disease
-Rrhea	flow or discharge
-Sphyxia	pulse
-Ema	condition
A-	without or no
Micro-	small
Brady-	slow

Practice Example 3

Write the medical word using the correct prefix/combining form/suffix for the following definitions

1. pertaining to the head	
2. painful digestion	

3. condition of scanty urine	
4. condition of two or more fingers joined together	
5. record of the heart's electrical activity	
6. surgical removal of the large intestine	
7. painful menstrual flow	
8. inflammation of the liver	
9. condition of blood, low sugar	
10. difficulty swallowing	

Answers: 1. cephalic, 2. dyspepsia, 3. Oliguria, 4. Syndactyly, 5. Electrocardiogram, 6. Colectomy, 7. Dysmenorrhea, 8. Hepatitis, 9. Hypoglycemia, 10. Dysphagia.

Practice Example 4

Write the meaning of the combining form

1. lumb/o	
2. mandibul/o	
3. ten/o	
4. derm/o	
5. xanth/o	
6. obsteter/o	

7. oste/o	
8. syncop/o	
9. vertigo/o	
10. chrom/o	

Answers: 1. lumbar region, lower back, 2. Jaw. 3. tendon, 4. Skin, 5. Yellow, 6. Pregnancy. 7. Bone, 8. To cut off or cut short, 9. Dizziness, 10. Color

Summary

While we have not completely exhausted the medical terminology dictionary, this chapter has given you a solid foundation on which you will continue to build throughout nursing school. Taking the time to learn how to break down a medical word, how to pronounce the word, and how to spell it will help you tremendously in both your nursing coursework and preparation for bedside clinical practice. Ensure that you are fully versed in each of the prefixes, suffixes, and combining forms presented in this chapter. Find additional medical words on your own and work to reveal their meaning using the techniques and tips in this chapter. Continue to practice using the online resources provided in this text as well as additional medical terminology websites and apps you may choose to download on an electronic device. Repetition and use will help prepare you for an incredible nursing career.

References

Bostwick, P. (2020). *Medical terminology: Learning through practice.* New York, NY: McGraw-Hill.

Chabner, D. E. (2015). *Medical terminology: A short course* (7th ed.). Maryland Heights, MO: Elsevier Saunders.

JaszLeo. (2018). Abbreviation. *Urban Dictionary.* Retrieved from https://www.urbandictionary.com/author.php?author=JaszLeo

Stedman's. (2014). *Stedman's medical abbreviations, acronyms & symbols* (5th ed.). New York, NY: Lippincott Williams & Wilkins.

Part 3: Nursing Calculations

Chapter 10

Introduction to Safe Nursing Practice

Chapter Objectives:

- Define a culture of safety in nursing.
- Understand the need for safety in nursing practice.
- Define the role of the Joint Commission, AHRQ, QSEN, and the IOM in safe nursing practice.
- Discuss ways in which nurses reduce medication errors.
- State the base six "rights" of safe medication administration.
- Define and discuss the value of medication reconciliation.

In general, nursing exists within what we refer to as a *culture of safety*. This means that safety is an integral part of who we are as nurses and the environment in which we choose to practice. It is infused into our patient care as well as our training. According to the American Nurses Association (2016), a culture of safety "describes the core values and behaviors that come about when there is a collective and continuous commitment by organizational leadership, manager, and health care workers to emphasize safety over competing goal" (para. 3). Safety as a culture ensures that everyone is involved and contributes to both personal, environmental, and patient safe practice. While entire books could be written, and in fact have been written, on the concepts of safety and quality, this brief chapter will introduce you to the basic fundamental principles involved in patient care, specifically directing your attention to the processes involved in delivering safe care rather than a discussion of personal or environmental practice. According to the Institute of Medicine (IOM) et al., patient safety is, "indistinguishable from the delivery of quality health care" (2004, p. 5).

In discussing this important topic, we must first look at the basic underlying definitions. The word safe refers to being, "secure from threat of danger, harm, or loss" (*Merriam-Webster*, 2020b, para. 1). It is described as an adjective and is generally associated with a behavior or action, such as seen in the following sentence: *the patient received safe nursing care*. Yet we find that the concept of safety seems vague and could mean "security from threat or danger" in really any situation. Specifically, what does it mean to be a *safe nurse* and *provide safe patient care*? Many independent agencies have attempted to define patient safety and safe nursing practice. Their exploration of the concepts and research think-tanks have led to more abstraction such as, prevent errors, or, build a culture of safety. Notice that the emphasis centers on action, meaning that safe nursing practice can be defined as "those [practices or actions] that reduce the risk of adverse events related to exposure to medical care across a range of diagnoses or condition" (AHRQ et al., 2001, p. 8). This definition means that there are specific evidence-based practices associated with safety in nursing that must be studied and applied to how nurses take care of patients every day.

Let us take a closer look at what quality refers to in a health care setting. Quality is "the standard of something as measured against other things of a similar kind; the degree of excellence of something" (*Merriam-Webster*, 2020a, para. 1). Despite the abstraction of these terms it is certainly evident that nursing has been concerned with practices that "reduce risk and adverse outcomes" and "measures of standards of excellence" since its inception. Did we not read in Chapter 2 that many great historical nursing figures worked tirelessly to improve the quality of care provided to patients through careful notation and deliberate nursing interventions? As safe nursing practice is directly linked to patient care quality, we should note that there is a well-established, positive relationship between the two concepts. As safe nursing practice increases, so does the quality of patient care.

AHRQ

The Agency for Healthcare Research and Quality (AHRQ) is a repository of data and evidence-based practices for all nurses and health care providers. This agency provides documented, well-researched, evidence-based practice guidelines. Safety is therefore built into every single nursing action and intervention performed by an RN including deciphering medical orders, preparing and administering medication.

JCAHO

Another independent agency at the forefront of safe nursing practice and quality patient care is the Joint Commission. Created by the Joint Commission, the current National Patient Safety Goals (NPSGs) became effective as of July 1, 2020, and are tailored to each health care sector. The 2020 Hospital National Patient Safety Goals include evidence-based actions that drastically reduce the likelihood of an error in patient care. These indicators provide guidance to nurses on current safety techniques and include:

- Identifying patients correctly (using at least two identifiers);
- Improving Staff Communication (providing important test results to the right person on time);
- Using medication safely (labeling medications that are not labeled, using caution with medicated patients, recording and passing along information about medicines correctly);
- Using alarms safely (making improvements to ensure alarms are audible and responded to timely);
- Preventing infection (using hand cleaning guidelines from the CDC and WHO and working to improve goals and outcomes);
- Identifying patient safety risks (reducing the risk for suicide); and finally
- Presenting mistakes in surgery (ensuring the correct surgery is done on the correct patient at the correct place, time, and body part, effectively using the concept of "time out") (The Joint Commission, 2020, p. 1).

QSEN

Quality and Safety Education for Nurses (QSEN) is an institute dedicated to your preparation, as student nurses for the future. They do this by providing core competencies for nursing practice to ensure safe quality nursing care. The QSEN competencies include competent: patient-centered care, teamwork and collaboration, use of evidence-based practice, use of data to ensure quality improvement, safety as a means of minimizing risk of harm, and the use of informatics for effective communication and error mitigation (QSEN, 2020). QSEN core competencies for safe and quality care can be downloaded by clicking the following link: https://drive.google.com/file/d/0B5YGF5c2vqn5cHFZcnZ5X09ST2s/edit

These are but a few of the numerous agencies focused on safe practice and quality patient care. From this information it should be quite clear that safety is one of nursing's most important goals and is based on careful, competent knowledge, skills acquisition, and professional attitudes. Let us next look at one of the most important roles of a nurse, the proper preparation and administration of medication.

Relationship of Medical Terminology to Safety

In our previous two chapters, we focused on learning the language of medicine and nursing. In this way nurses must understand the language of health care to ensure safe care practices. Let us use the following written order, for a medication, as an example. In the following image, what does the prescription say? As a nurse, if you cannot read the order, how can you ensure that you are giving the correct medication?

The medication being ordered in the image indicates Glucophage XL, a medication for diabetes mellitus. Can you tell what the dose says? Does it say 50 mg or 500 mg or 50 mcg? Even the smallest error in administering the wrong amount of a medication can be devastating to a patient's outcome. How often should the medication be given? Does it say give 2 pills by mouth every day or perhaps two pills by mouth every other day? Safe medication administration and nursing practice involves ensuring that everyone on the team is working together on behalf of the patient. In the beginning of this chapter, we discussed evidence-based practices that help ensure safety. Organizations focused on safety and quality, have helped everyone in health care realize that there are some basic steps that can easily be accomplished. These safety measures have included: (1) The use of electronic systems to enter and manage medication orders. Instead of handwritten orders, medical providers are being required, when available, to use a computer and an electronic medical record, to type medication and other patient care orders. (2) Additional safety precautions include involving the users of patient care systems in designing and developing electronic health recording systems. The need for nurses to work with information technology specialists has created a nursing role as a nursing informatics expert. The role of this person is to ensure that all nursing related documentation systems are easily accessible and reflect the correct assessments and documentation required by nurses. It would be a significant mistake to allow people who do not understand the needs and requirements of nursing practice to design workflow documents, as this could potentially increase errors and negatively impact patient safety. User-centered designs make items clear and easy to find. They also make it more difficult for nurses to skip steps or find a "work-around" ensuring safe nursing practice and standardized processes. One of the most significant contributions to user-centered process design has been fail safe features built into medication records. Nurses can become extremely busy. A built-in safeguard requires nurses to stop and double check medications, orders, amounts and other important criteria, such as allergies. A double-check prompt, built into an electronic medical record, will not allow a nurse to administer a medication without a second verification entered in the system by a different RN. Additional safeguard prompts require the RN to enter a lab value or a vital sign before being able to access or give a specific amount of medication. (3) RNs frequently need to document patient care. Often, RNs need to move from room to room before having time to chart patient information. It is easy for RNs to confuse patient information because they are relying on their memory of an event or a specific time and they are waiting to document findings. The third patient safety technique streamlines processes and documentation so that RNs have the ability to immediately chart a finding or record a value in a patient's room, in lieu of waiting to return to the nursing station and find an open computer. (4) Safety also means involving the patients in their own care. By including patients and families directly in their care, nurses can ensure correct and accurate histories, correct medication dosages, and better access to patient medical information through patient portal systems.

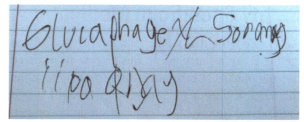

Writing example provided by Alex Hopersberger. Reprinted by permission.

	Definitions in Patient Safety
Side-effect:	A known effect, other than that primarily intended, relating to the pharmacological properties of a medication. Example: an opiate analgesia causes nausea.
Adverse reaction:	Unexpected harm arising from a justified action where the correct process was followed for the context in which the event occurred. Example: an unexpected allergic reaction in a patient taking a medication for the first time.
Error:	Failure to carry out a planned action as intended or application of an incorrect plan.
Adverse event:	An incident in which a patient is harmed.

Source: World Health Organization. (2020). *Patient Safety: Topic 11, improving medication safety.* Retrieved from https://www.who.int/patientsafety/education/curriculum/PSP_mpc_topic-11.pdf

Safety Specific to Medication Administration

Acknowledging that medication safety is a significant topic in health care requires that each clinician standardize medication practices. In this text we have already learned the importance of high-level critical thinking in nursing practice. Let us put critical thinking together now with the concept of medication administration. Recall that critical thinking is a process of thought that involves reasonable and rational action. As such, it requires foundational knowledge, organization skills, competency of technique, autonomy, attention to detail, and clinical reasoning. The nurse's role therefore in preventing medication errors includes ensuring open communication with patients and other members of the health care team. The nurse's second role in preventing medication errors involves reporting medication errors when they occur to the agency risk management department. Nurses do not regard reporting errors of any kind as a punitive process. Remember the RN's duty to patients is through honesty and beneficence. Nurses view error reporting as a positive practice which is valued in discovering higher level errors that may involve more than just the nurse on one particular floor or department. When everyone reports a problem, the risk management department has the opportunity to look for trends and determine root causes. This is what is meant by quality management and assurance: working every day to do our best as a team to improve patient care. The third role of the nurse in preventing medication errors is to always adhere to safety standards. Standards set by agencies like The Joint Commission help hospitals identify common trends and improve patient care. These safety initiatives such as the use of new technology, reduces human error and improves quality. Fourth, nurses and providers alike are encouraged to always use generic names with medication, unless a brand is required to standardize language. Fifth, nurses are also encouraged to recognize high-risk, sound alike, look-alike medication names and packaging to avoid potential error. Sixth, nurses are trained to involve the patient in medication administration to help reduce errors. Patients know what medications they take, what they look like, and when they should be administered. Partnering with the patient to ensure they know exactly what they are receiving, when, and why helps to reduce potential errors. Lastly, follow the JCAHO "Do Not Use" guidelines which include avoiding errors in writing medication doses. This means, avoiding the use of a training zero when writing any number, especially as it applies to indicating the strength or amount of a medication: example, write 1 not 1.0 to avoid the entry appearing as a 10 instead of as a 1. Similarly, always use a leading zero in front of a decimal point to indicate that the amount prescribed accurately reflects a portion of a whole number. For example, write 0.1 instead of simply .1 to ensure clarity. Note that .1 without a preceding zero can easily be misinterpreted as 1. Finally, if one cannot use an electronic medical record for clear entries of medications, ensure that you transcribe or write verbal orders from providers neatly, printing clearly.

Safe Medication Administration: The Six Rights

Within nursing, there are six "rights" or "safety checks" that must be performed to ensure we do not inadvertently cause an error in administering a medication to a patient. Although we are capable of human error, nurses are held to much higher standards for good reason. Remember the ethical principles of nursing? What does the principle of nonmaleficence mean? Nonmaleficence means "do no harm." The American Nurses Association Code of Ethics contains numerous statements that specifically apply to medication administration and are summarized below:

1. The nurse acts to safeguard the patient from incompetent, unethical, or illegal practice.
2. The nurse assumes responsibility and accountability for nursing judgments and actions.
3. The nurse maintains competence in nursing.

These standards involve autonomy (the right of the patient to be informed about medications and the right to refuse medications), truthfulness (the nurse has the obligation not to lie, this includes not concealing an action or not disclosing information with regard to informed consent with medication trials), beneficence (the nurse will always act in the patient's best interest), nonmaleficence (the nurse will never cause a patient harm and must prevent harm whenever possible), confidentiality (the nurse must respect and keep in confidence any information, including the types of medication a patient may be taking from those who do not need to know), justice (this refers to the patient's right to receive the right drug, the right dose, via the correct route and at the right time), and fidelity (the nurse has the obligation to keep promises).

Remembering our ethical principles while performing all roles in nursing practice requires nurses to develop safe standardized processes. One example of a safe process was the creation of the six rights of safe medication of administration provided below. The six rights include:

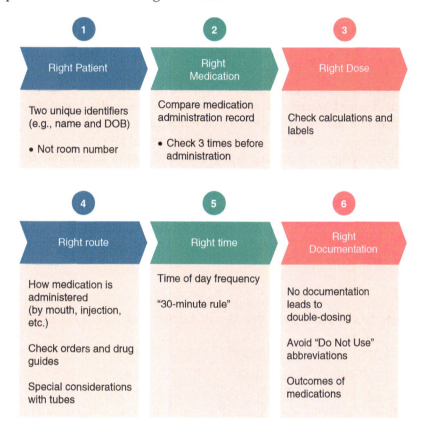

Other "Rights" of the patient involve:

- The right indication: This means that the patient understands the reason for a medication being ordered and administered.
- The right to know. Nurses are responsible to educate patients regarding all prescribed medications.
- The right to refuse. Patients cannot be made to take medications except in extreme circumstances. These circumstances may include a court order, a dangerous patient, or Kendra's Law. If a patient refuses an ordered medication, it is the responsibility of the nurse to document the patient's refusal and notify caregiver that the medication was not provided to the patient as ordered.

Watch the following quick video Picmonic on *The Six Rights of Medication* to help you remember the components: https://www.picmonic.com/share/picmonic/6-rights-of-medication-administration_1507?browse=null&browseParams=%7B%7D&browseOptions=%7B%22open%22:false%7D?utm_source=generic&utm_medium=social&utm_term=1463760192&utm_content=text_link&utm_campaign=player_share_link&ref=GC73N0ZJOKLZLFM20

Medication Reconciliation and Safe Practice

Medication reconciliation is the process of comparing medications the patient has been taking at home with the medications a patient is prescribed while in a hospital or other health care setting. Why might this be an important safety consideration? On admission, nurses need to get a thorough history of current medications.

Have you ever been asked by a doctor's office or nurse in a hospital to bring in your medications or to bring a list of current medications? This process of accurately verifying your home medications was developed to provide safety. When patients are in distress, they often forget what medications they are on or omit important aspects of how they take their medication. This is a common concern for many people. Have you ever been asked what the name of the medication you take every day is? Can you remember all of the details? Most often nurses encounter patients who make statements like, "I don't remember....it starts with an M and it's small and green in color." Can you tell what medication the patient is referring to? Nurses use medication reconciliation to: (1) ensure that the same medications can be given to the patient that are being taken at home, (2) new medications can be written and providers can avoid any potential complications that may arise from medication interactions, (3) the exact amount of medication is known for providers to make decisions regarding the dosage. Imagine being on a critical medication, like insulin at home. You are admitted to the hospital and the nurse asks you what medications you currently take each day. If you are confused because you have actually been admitted for low blood sugar, you may not remember the name, strength, or amount of the medication you take before each meal. When we look at the potential for error in this situation, it is high. As a student, if you did not know, there are six main types of insulin. Insulin is critical to the body as it regulates blood sugar. If your body is not producing enough and you depend on insulin every day, critical patient safety errors can be made when the proper medication and amount is not accurately maintained from one setting to another. The value of medication reconciliation is that nurses can avoid many forms of medication errors which may include transcribing medications, omissions of medications, duplication of therapy and potential medication interactions.

Chapter Video

Take a moment to watch, *Beyond The Bedside: The Nurse's Role in Quality, Safety and Service.*
https://youtu.be/4UUSZjoeo4I

Summary

Nursing embraces a culture of safety in every aspect of its role. Safe nursing practice and quality of patient care have a positive relationship. As safe practice increases so does patient care quality. Organizations and agencies such as IOM, AHRQ, JCAHO, and QSEN help establish safe practice standards and work to reduce error. There are numerous evidence-based strategies in place to assist nurses and health care workers in ensuring safe practices including during the administration of patient medications. Remembering the ethical principles that apply to all nursing situations and developing repetitious safety habits such as adherence to the six patient medication rights of administration will greatly reduce the chance for medication error. Taking safety seriously and knowing your responsibilities for safe nursing practice will result in improved patient outcomes.

References

Agency for Healthcare Research and Quality [AHRQ], Shojania, K. G., Duncan, B. W., McDonald, K. M., et al., (Eds.). (2001). *Making health care safer: A critical analysis of patient safety practices Evidence Report/Technology Assessment No 43* (Prepared by the University of California at San Francisco-Stanford Evidence-based Practice Center under Contract No 290-97-0013) AHRQ Publication No. 01-E058. Retrieved from https://www.ncbi.nlm.nih.gov/books/NBK11945/?report=printable

Institute of Medicine (US) Committee on Data Standards for Patient Safety, Aspden, P., Corrigan, J. M., Wolcott, J., & Erickson, S. M. (Eds.). (2004). *Patient Safety: Achieving a New Standard for Care.* National Academies Press (US). Retrieved from https://www.ncbi.nlm.nih.gov/books/NBK216086/pdf/Bookshelf_NBK216086.pdf

Le, J. (2019). Drug administration. *MSD Manual Online.* Retrieved from https://www.msdmanuals.com/en-kr/home/drugs/administration-and-kinetics-of-drugs/drug-administration

Merriam-Webster. (2020a). Quality. *Merriam-Webster.com dictionary*. Retrieved from https://www.merriam-webster.com/dictionary/quality

Merriam-Webster. (2020b). Safe. *Merriam-Webster.com dictionary*. Retrieved from https://www.merriam-webster.com/dictionary/safe

Shepherd, M., & Shepherd, E. (2020). Medicines administration 1: Understanding routes of administration. *Nursing Times* [online], *116*(6), 42–44. Retrieved from https://www.nursingtimes.net/clinical-archive/medicine-management/medicines-administration-1-understanding-routes-of-administration-24-04-2020/

The Joint Commission. (2020). *Hospital: National Patient Safety Goals*. Retrieved from https://www.jointcommission.org/standards/national-patient-safety-goals/hospital-2020-national-patient-safety-goals/

Chapter 11

Introduction to Medication Administration

> **Chapter Objectives:**
> - Identify factors that influence medication dosages.
> - Identify the common routes for medication administration.
> - Identify the components of a medication order.
> - Identify meanings of standard abbreviations used in medication administration.
> - Interpret a given medication order.
> - Identify the location of the trade and generic names of medications on a label.
> - Identify the dosage strength of medications.
> - Identify the forms in which a medication is supplied and administered.

Despite having had years of math education, many people who are interested in becoming a nurse often share that math and math courses cause a sense of apprehension and anxiety when reviewing nursing school requirements. How much math do nurses use? Can you be successful? in this chapter, you will be introduced to medical math and the equipment used for medication administration. Nurses use math every single day and with every single patient encounter. Although the level of math required for nursing school is generally limited to basic algebra, it is imperative that student nurses become fully competent in math calculations given the high-stake nature of their role in patient care and medication administration. Let us begin with an introduction to the common routes for medication administration.

Common Routes for Medication Administration

According to Le (2019), a medication route refers to the path in which a medication or other substance is administered into the body and are commonly classified by location. When defining a route of administration by location, there are over 100 routes identified. Each route has a specific purpose, advantage and disadvantage (FDA, 2017). See: https:// www.fda.gov/drugs/data-standards-manual-monographs/route-administration

According to Shepherd and Shepherd (2020), there are three main categories of medication administration. These categories follow nursing's traditional definition of route, which is not centered in the application point of entry as noted by Le (2019) and the FDA (2017) but rather with regard to how a medication enters the body.

1. **Enteral Administration Routes**: Defined as an oral (PO) route containing any of the following additional oral methods.
    a. Sublingual (SL) (under the tongue),
    b. Buccal (in the mouth along the inside of the cheek), or via
    c. Enteral feeding tube (a tube that is inserted to the level of the stomach or small intestine).

2. **Parenteral Administration Routes**: Defined as a direct injection into the body, this route contains all of the following methods.
   a. Intravenous (IV)
   b. Intramuscular (IM)
   c. Subcutaneous (SQ)
   d. Intradermal (ID)
3. **Topical Administration Routes**: Defined as a route in which medication is applied directly to skin or mucosa; there are aaseveral subcategories of this route that are specific to how a medication is best absorbed. These methods include:
   a. Transdermal (topically applied medicated patch or disc);
   b. Instillation (such as an eye, nose, or ear drop);
   c. Inhalation (INH) (such as an inhaler to get medication directly into the lungs);
   d. Insertion (Supp) (such as a suppository for the rectum or vagina) (p. 42).

As a student nurse, it is imperative to understand that the route of administration of a medication is predetermined by the manufacturer. If a patient cannot tolerate a medication, for instance if a patient cannot swallow a tablet, then an alternative route can only be used under the direction of a prescribing provider. Medications cannot be exchanged for a different form, such as from a tablet to a liquid form, without the original medication order being cancelled and a new order for the same medication, in the alternate form, written by the prescribing provider. Registered Nurses do not have prescriptive authority and can therefore not make this determination under their scope of practice. This is another reason why effective communication and teamwork is an essential component of patient care.

Equipment Needed for Oral Medication Administration

Note the following images. The first image shows an opaque palm-sized medicine cup that is used to provide liquid medication to patients in standard measurements of mL (as shown) and on the reverse side of the cup, in teaspoon and tablespoon calibrations. A medication cup holds up to 30 mL which is equivalent to 1 fluid oz. or 2 tablespoons. You will refresh your knowledge of conversion tables in the upcoming chapters.

In the second image, a small white paper cup is shown. This small white cup is called a Soufflé cup and is used for solids such as tablets or capsules. It is an unacceptable practice for nurses to place medications directly into the hand of a patient. Medications can easily become contaminated or dropped when using this method and should therefore always be placed in a clean disposable Soufflé cup. The cup is then handed to the patient for self-administration.

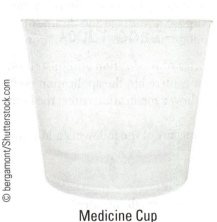
Medicine Cup

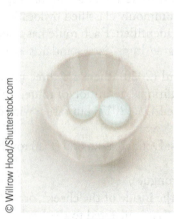
Soufflé Cup

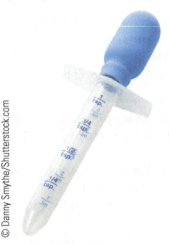
Calibrated Dropper

The final image shows a calibrated dropper. A calibrated dropper is used to administer small amounts of liquid medication often to children. Note that the dropper can be calibrated in milliliters as well as in teaspoons. These small amounts correspond to the amounts given to children as pediatric medications are always based on the weight of the child.

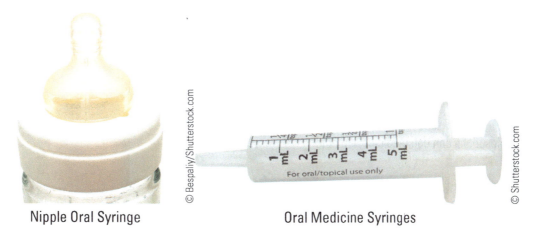

Nipple Oral Syringe   **Oral Medicine Syringes**

The image above and the one to the left are photos of two different types of oral syringes.

An oral syringe is used to administer oral medications to those who may not be able to swallow medications in solid forms, such as a pill or capsule. This may include young children as well as older adults. Additionally, an oral syringe may be dark in color (not pictured) which is intentional and is selected by the nurse for use with orally administered liquid medications that may react to direct light exposure. The dark color provides a shield from UV light much like that of a pair of sunglasses for the eyes. The other oral syringe is clear and can be used with any oral liquid medication. Note that both oral syringes have a limit to the amount of medication they can hold. In the image displayed, the nurse would only select the oral syringe if the liquid volume of medication ordered was less than or equal to 5 mL or two teaspoons.

The image to the left of the oral syringes is that of a nipple. Notice that the nipple is part of a white lid. The nipple shown here is the top component of a baby bottle. Notice that the nipple is not calibrated like the oral syringe or medication cup. The use of the nipple in oral medication administration is simply the means by which the medication is provided to the infant. All medications would first be drawn up in a syringe to ensure proper volume and then directly administered into the nipple while the infant is sucking. The use of the nipple in medication administration forms a safe method for newborns and infants who are still primarily feeding from a standard breast milk or formula bottle.

Reading a Meniscus

Reading a medication cup, when it contains a liquid medication, involves understanding how to interpret the meniscus. According to *Merriam-Webster* (2020), a meniscus refers to "the curved upper surface of a column of liquid" (para 1). Look at the image. Note the curved shape to the liquid. Given the presence of the liquid, it is important to realize that the amount being measured in the cup is determined by looking at the bottom, middle portion of the curve. In the following image, the amount in the medication cup represents 2 tsp or 10 mL. Note that the sides of the liquid curve slightly on the sides. This is not the location from which to interpret the volume. Additionally, when reading any liquid medication, one of the most significant considerations is to ensure that you are looking at the amount or volume of medication in the cup from eye level. If you try to read the volume in the cup from any other angle, the

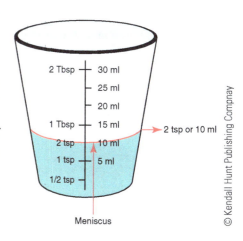

meniscus will appear to shift and cause an error in determining the true volume. Always place the medication cup on a flat surface and then bend down to ensure the meniscus is at eye level before interpreting the volume.

Practice Example 1

Take a moment and challenge your comprehension. Can you answer the following questions?

Which device can you use to administer 1.5 mL of an oral medication?
How many tablespoons can one medicine cup hold?
Differentiate between the sublingual and buccal routes of administration.
What should you do if you make a med error?
Discuss some special considerations for a pediatric or geriatric patient.

Answers: 1) Oral syringe, 2) 2 Tbs, 3) Sublingual (SL)—placed under tongue; buccal—placed in mouth against cheek, 4) Continually assess the patient, inform the physician, and document per agency policy. 5) a) In the geriatric population, two thirds use Rx and OTC meds. Physiologic changes in an older adult involves a slowing of function: changes in circulation, absorption, metabolism, excretion, and stress response. Geriatric patients have a lowered body mass and can have changes in mental status when dosed with the wrong amount of a medication. Geriatric patients require lower doses than adults, as a rule and may need special delivery devices, visual aid to read labels, and easy-open lids. Allow extra time for teaching; clients should demonstrate back what you taught them. b) In the pediatric population, medication is ALWAYS based on the infant or child's weight. As medications are new to this population, careful observation of an infant or child is required. Medications are often liquid and are flavored to increase palatability so ensuring medications are safely stored using child proof containers and locks is essential.

Let us now turn our attention to the components of a medication order. In previous chapters, we have learned medical abbreviations, communication strategies, and medical terminology. Understanding how a medication order is structured and what is involved in medication orders will help you work as a team to ensure orders are clear and appropriate before administering the medication.

The Components of a Medication Order

Understanding an Order

The RN cannot generate a medical order of any kind. An RN may only receive a medical order and transcribe the order for direct patient care. A medical order refers to a legal direction of care or treatment by a specifically identified provider, that may or may not include a medication. The provision of all medical orders is beyond the scope of the Registered Nurse and is illegal.

Prior to implementation, a legal *written* order or prescription from a health care provider is required. Notice that the word "written" in the last sentence is italicized. Current safety guidelines require orders to be clearly written or typed electronically for safety. We will review the very specific conditions in which a verbal order may be given in the next section.

There are various types of medical orders.

A medical "order set" or "order sheet" as described below, resembles the following:

Patient Full Name, Date of Birth, Medical Record Number, Date/Time

1. Admit to the medical-surgical inpatient unit.
2. Activity: Bed rest with bathroom privileges.
3. Vital signs: q4h and as needed; call for temperature greater than 101° F, pulse less than 60, BP less than 80/40 or greater than 150/90.
4. Diet: 1,800 cal ADA.
5. Strict I/Os.
6. Furosemide 20mg po qAM.
7. Start 18g IV to saline lock.
8. Labs: CBC, Chem12 stat; call with results.
9. IV fluid: 0.9% NS to run at 1,000 mL/8 hr

The above set of order would then be signed by the ordering provider.

In the following table, the type of order followed by an example is provided for your review. Notice that each type of order is used in specific situations and that some types involve a group of orders rather than a single order.

	Types of Provider Orders
Standing order: Routine order	A standing order is an order that is used by a provider for a condition as a matter of routine. For instance, a provider may admit patient for a specific surgery and, unless allergic to the medication, will provide the patient with a course of antibiotics. Example: Ampicillin 1 g IV q6h for 4 doses
Prn order: administered as needed	A prn order is a medical order that allows a patient to have a specific treatment as needed or desired under certain circumstance without having to call the provider for each request. Example: Tylenol 650mg po q4h prn for temp greater than 101° F
Stat order: administered immediately	A stat order requires an immediate action by the RN. Example: Ativan 2mg IM stat
Single (one-time) order: administered only once	A single order reflects the administration or completion of a therapy once. Example: Tdap 0.5mL IM × 1
"Provider's 'Order Set' or 'Order Sheet'"	A list of orders written by the provider which may include several medications and general care orders. This order sheet, meaning usually a full page of instructions, is then noted by nurse and "unit clerk or secretary."

Part of the RN's role with a written order and a paper chart is to transcribe all medication orders onto the Medication Administration Record (MAR) after faxing the order sheet to the pharmacy. In health care facilities with electronic medical records, orders are entered by the provider electronically, verified by the nurse, and transmitted onto the electronic medication administration record. The pharmacy then verifies the medication orders and sends the ordered medication, at the correct intervals, to the location of the patient. The nurse who administers a medication is accountable for all consequences and reactions a patient may experience if an error is made, regardless of who transcribes the medication to the MAR. Nurses are required to double check all orders and compare the MAR to the medication order as well as directly to the medication sent to be administered from the pharmacy. Recall in the previous chapter that several standardized safety practices have been developed to ensure patient safety and nurse compliance. It is the RNs duty and obligation to the patient (do no harm) that holds the RN responsible in all circumstances.

Verbal Orders

Verbal orders are orders obtained orally from the provider to the RN. They occur directly from a provider to the nurse and can be obtained by telephone or in person. Recall that our chapters on communication and safety discussed the potential danger associated with this type of order. Orders can be easily heard incorrectly for numerous reasons including background noise, distraction, rate of speech, lack of tone or use of inflection, or hearing loss, to name a few. Because of new safety standards, it is no longer acceptable to use a verbal order as a common ordering method. The use of a verbal order may only be used during an emergency situation by qualified staff. As a standardized safe practice, the RN should always follow the following guideline: *WRITE it, READ it back, receive CONFIRMATION*. This means the RN must immediately write down what was stated by the provider, read it back to the provider exactly as it is written, and wait until the provider confirms the order is correct before proceeding. The prescribing provider is then required to sign the order, either on the written order or electronically, within 24 hours. It is well documented that errors may be prevented by using computerized physician order entry or fax transmissions in all situations.

Writing Medication Orders

The nurse should be aware that there are 7 *ESSENTIAL* components of all medication orders. In fact, an order is not complete and therefore cannot be implemented unless all seven components are present. The essential components of a medication order are:

1. **Client's *full* name:** The order must be directly linked to a specific patient. In electronic charting, a patient's record must be entered before any orders can be made, thus ensuring the identification of the patient.
2. **Date and time written:** An order must be dated and timed. An entry must detail when an order was written because some orders may expire and/or orders are recorded from oldest to most recent. For instance, if a medication is ordered for 3 days, how would you know when the medication should end if you did not know when it was originally ordered?
3. **Name of medication:** The generic name of the medication is required unless a brand name is specifically ordered for the medical benefit of the exact brand medication.
4. **Dosage:** The dosage refers to the quantity and strength of the medication such as 50 mg or 3 tsp.
5. **Route:** The route, as learned earlier refers to the way in which the medication will be given
6. **Time and frequency:** The time and frequency refer to how often the medication will be given and taken
7. **Signature of prescriber or proxy:** Only the person prescribing the medication may sign the order. A nurse, as a proxy, may sign an order only as an acknowledgement of receipt of the order but cannot by scope of practice directly order any medication.

Interpreting a Medication Order

If parts are missing—the order is NOT legal and should NOT be completed!

As a nurse you will be responsible to ensure that all medication orders can be clearly understood. If, for any reason, an order is unclear the RN must stop and clarify the order with the prescribing provider. An order, as noted previously must be written in a specific order and contain specific components. Note the components and sequence of a properly written medication order in the following the adjacent diagram.

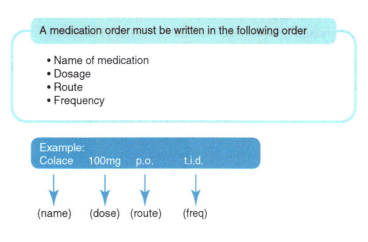

Note the specific sequence to the order as shown in the diagram. If a component of any medication order is missing, it will then be easily identified. This is another example of a standardized safe practice in health care.

Never Assume— Clarify the Order if In Doubt!

Practice Example 2

For each medication listed here, organize the medication orders in the correct sequence:

25mg PR Phenergan b.i.d.
Zofran ODT prn nausea q4hr 8mg SL
IV Reglan once 10mg
Daily p.o. Meclazine 25mg

Answers: 1) Phenergan 25mg PR b.i.d. 2) Zofran ODT 8mg SL q4hrs prn nausea 3) Reglan 10mg IV once 4) Meclazine 25mg p.o. daily

Special Considerations in Writing an Order

There are a few special considerations that may apply when writing a medication order. The route is VERY important as the mechanism of action of any medication is directly related to the route of administration. Administering a medication without first clarifying the exact route could be very dangerous to the health of your patient. For instance, medications intended for intravenous or intramuscular injection could be poisonous or completely ineffective if administered as an oral liquid medication. Never assume you know the route. Clarify and double check all medication information. Secondly, the frequency of a medication can change, if the facility has a standardized time in which medications are given to patients. Therefore, if it is important to the effectiveness of the medication or treatment to always clarify the frequency, especially when working in an agency with standardized abbreviations and time ranges. Finally, sometimes medications come with special instructions. These special instructions can easily be overlooked in a medication order as they routinely come after the standard nomenclature. These special instructions can mean everything to the safety of your patient and the potential for medication error. Special instructions can include statements such as, "hold if….," give ½ hour before …," and, "for blood pressure greater than…" In instances like these, special instructions should always be highlighted, enlarged, or emboldened.

Interpreting Prescription Orders Containing Abbreviations

Recall from the chapter on abbreviations that several of the abbreviations were associated with time and route. Both forms of abbreviations can be found in a single medication order. Take a moment to review the time and route abbreviations in the following table to ensure your familiarity.

Abbreviation	Meaning	Example	Do NOT Use
ac	Before meals	Up to 30 minutes before the patient eats (7:30 a.m. for a patient who will begin eating breakfast at 8 a.m.)	
pc	After meals	Up to 30 minutes after the patient eats (12:30 p.m. for a patient who finished lunch at 12 noon)	
daily	Every day	Every day at 8 a.m.	DO NOT USE qd or q.d.
bid	Twice a day	Evenly spread in two 12-hour periods (8 a.m. and again at 8 p.m.)	
tid	Three times a day	Evenly spread in three 8-hour periods (midnight, 8 a.m. and 4 p.m.)	
qid	Four times a day	Evenly spread in four 6-hour periods (midnight, 6 a.m., 12 noon, 6 p.m.)	
qh	Every hour	Giving the medication every hour or 24 times in one day	
At bedtime	At the hour of sleep	Given at the time the patient normally goes to sleep (your patient tells you he goes to bed at 10 p.m., so the medication is set for 10 p.m.)	DO NOT USE hs or h.s.
qn	Every night	Given after 7 p.m. but with no specified time such as at 10 p.m. The patient may take it as scheduled by the facility between 7 p.m. and midnight.	
stat	Immediately	This word means right now. If the provider orders the medication stat the nurse has within 5 minutes to administer the medication but no longer.	
every other day	Every other day	Taking a medication in a way that alternates days, usually at the same time on each of the days. (the medication is given at 8 a.m. on a Monday, Wed, Fri, Sunday schedule, and then Tues, Thurs, Saturday and so on).	DO NOT USE qod or q.o.d
prn	As directed or as needed	This abbreviation is always accompanied by a specific time interval and the indication for administration (Tylenol 325mg po q6h prn mild discomfort)	
Write out the words: Right ear/eye	Right ear/eye	Medication or lubricant placed in the right eye or ear using a dropper or small eye drop bottle	DO NOT USE AD/OD

Abbreviation	Meaning	Example	Do NOT Use
Write out the words: Left ear/eye	Left ear/eye	Medication or lubricant placed in the left eye or ear using a dropper or small eye drop bottle	DO NOT USE AL/OS
Write out the words: Each ear/eye	Each ear/eye	Medication or lubricant placed in the both eyes or ears using a dropper or small eye drop bottle	DO NOT USE AU/OU
IM	Intramuscularly	This is an injection, at a 90-degree angle, given into the muscle	
IV	Intravenously	Fluid medication or maintenance fluid, instilled directly into the vein through a plastic cannula and tubing that is continuously flowing at a specified rate	
IVPB	Intravenous piggyback	Fluid medication prepared in a separate small amount of fluid that is connected directly to the tube of the IV line and instilled into the vein at specific times.	
MDI	Metered dose inhaler	This is an aerosol device which delivers medication by inhalation into the lungs	
NGT or ng	Nasogastric tube	Medication is crushed or liquefied and instilled into the stomach or small intestine through a tube inserted in the nose which descends down the nasopharynx and ends in the ordered location (stomach or small intestine).	
po or PO	Orally or by mouth	The medication is given by mouth to the patient but may include any oral form such as a tablet, liquid, capsule that is swallowed	
pr or PR	Per rectum	The medication is prepared in a suppository form for easy absorption and inserted directly into the rectum of the patient	
Write out the word: Sub q or subcutaneously	Subcutaneously	The medication is placed in a special subcutaneous syringe and injected under the skin into the subcutaneous tissue via a 45 degree angle.	DO NOT USE sc, sq, s.c, or s.q
SL	Sublingual or under the tongue	The medication will disintegrate and absorb directly into the patient's system when placed under the tongue.	
ID	Intradermally	The medication is placed in a special tuberculin syringe and injected under the skin but above the subcutaneous tissue via a 5 to 15 degree angle.	

Interpreting Medication Labels

The next part of understanding the basics of medication administration involves understanding how to properly read a medication label. First it is important to understand that there are two general classifications of drugs: prescription only (Rx only) and over-the-counter (OTC).

In this section we will review each component of the label and compare prescription medication labels for multiple drugs to those that can be purchased "over the counter" or without a prescription on the common shelves of any drug or convenience store. Let us begin by first learning the parts of every medication label.

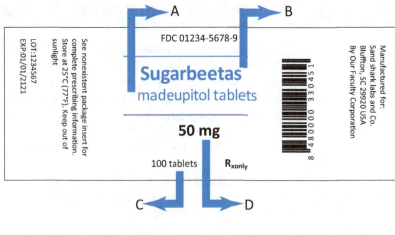

A generic name (madeupitol)   B trade name (Sugarbeetas)
C amount and form (100 tablets) D dosage strength (50mg)

In the given label, note the complexity. A significant amount of information is present on every label, intentionally. While this may appear a bit overwhelming initially, the safe care of patients extends to the Food and Drug Administration (FDA) and their oversight on all medications produced in the United States. The role of the FDA is to ensure that each medication label contains all the required information; they are also the regulatory agency in charge of monitoring the safe and proper creation, storage, and quality of the medication identified on the label. As you may be aware, medications produced in other countries may not have the same strict guidelines for medication production and distribution. In addition to the components listed in the given label from A through D, note the Lot number section and Expiration date. This is a required component of every medication and it is unethical for facilities to use medications that have expired. Medication may not be as effective past the date of expiration. Additionally, if a medication is taken off the market (what is referred to as a *recall*), for any reason, the lot number will be used to identify all involved products.

Let us now learn how to read a medication label by breaking it down into manageable parts. We begin with reading a generic medication label. A generic medication, according to the FDA (2018), refers to a medication created to be the same as an existing approved brand-name drug in dosage, form, safety, strength, route of administration, quality, and performance characteristics" (Generic drug facts, para 1).

Reading the Label: Generic Names

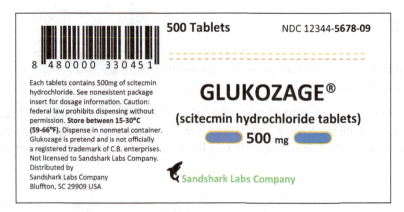

Glukozage label. Notice the two names. The first, *Glukozage*, is the trade name, identified by the registration symbol®. The name in smaller and different print is *scitecmin hydrochloride,* the generic or official name.

Generic names of medications are:

	Given by manufacturer who develops the med
	Not capitalized and refer to all medications in the category despite brand name
	Legally required on all labels
	Required to be known along with the brand or trade name, by all RNs
	Dispensed less expensively than brand
	Commonly used by providers. Examples include: morphine, atropine, furosemide, meperidine
	A reason for potential error as some generics Look-alike and their names may sound-alike—very different, use "Tall-man" letters: busPIRone vs buPROPion

Look at the labels carefully to ensure you become familiar with generic labels and their components.

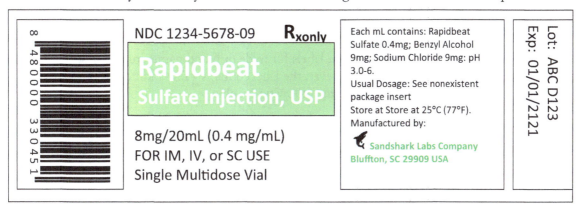

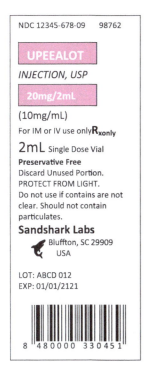

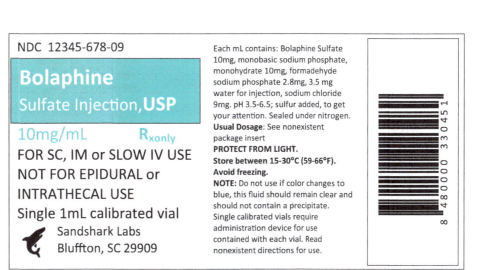

150 Chapter 11 Introduction to Medication Administration

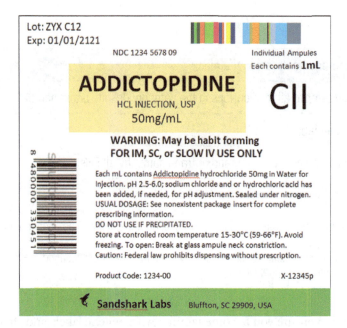

Reading the Label: Trade Name

Now let us look at a few examples of medication labels for trade or brand name drugs. These medications are also only available by provider prescription; however, the label contains a few additional components not provided on a generic label. Note the difference in the following graphic.

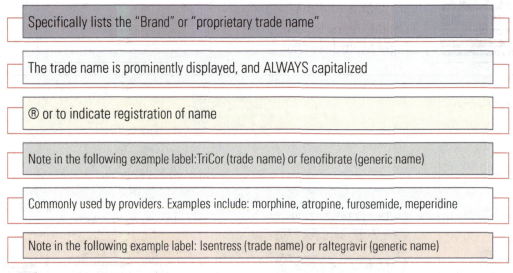

- Specifically lists the "Brand" or "proprietary trade name"
- The trade name is prominently displayed, and ALWAYS capitalized
- ® or to indicate registration of name
- Note in the following example label: TriCor (trade name) or fenofibrate (generic name)
- Commonly used by providers. Examples include: morphine, atropine, furosemide, meperidine
- Note in the following example label: Isentress (trade name) or raltegravir (generic name)

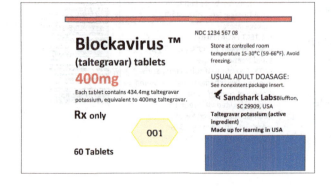
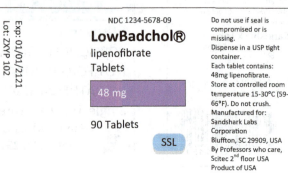

What is different about the above labels as compared to the generic labels? Do you see the image of the pill on both labels? Trade or brand name prescription medication also has a registered color and shape with a very specific stamp on each medication. In fact, if you find a medication on a floor table and you want to know what it is, you can look up a medication on the internet using the shape, color, and information stamped on the pill as identifiers.

Reading the Label: Dosage Strength

When it comes to reading the dosage strength on a label, you will notice three key features.

Weight or amount of medication provided in a specific unit of measure	• Solid meds = amount of med per tab, cap, etc. • e.g., amoxicillin 250 mg per capsule • Liquid meds = amount of med per mL, L, etc. • e.g., lactulose 10 g per 15 mL
Dosage strength may be stated in two different but equivalent dosage strengths	• e.g., Forteo 0.25 mg per mL = 250 mcg per mL
Dosage strength is sometimes expressed as a ratio or percent	• e.g., epinephrine 1 g per 1,000 mL (1:1000)

Do not let the dosage strength confuse you. As you continue your education and training in nursing the dosage strength will become familiar as the name of a medication becomes familiar. The chemical composition of medications dictates the units of measure for dosage strength. With repetition of use you will come to understand the dosage strength of every medication as well as the route and any special considerations required in its administration. Note the following examples of medications whose dosage strength is provided in both a ratio form and as a percentage.

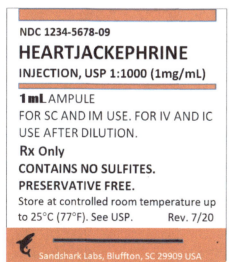
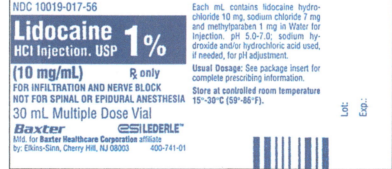

Reading the Label: Form

The form refers to how the medication is supplied: a tablet, capsule, liquid, and so forth. It is the type of medication found in the package. Each form of medication has specific rules for administration and may also require special handling. One such rule involves the administration of a capsule.

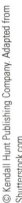
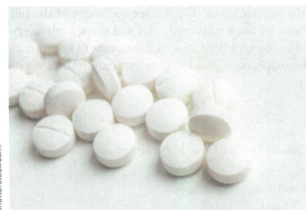
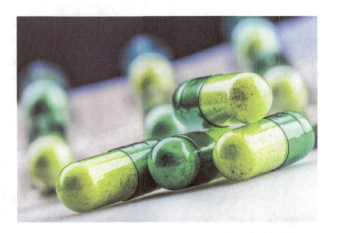

While a tablet may be crushed and is often scored (a tablet with an indented line down the middle as shown in the preceding image) so that it could be easily split in half, a capsule cannot be crushed or split into pieces. This is because a capsule generally contains a medication requiring the tiny beads or powder form of the medication contained within the capsule to be released over time or allowed to be slowly added to the body in a specific digestive location. Note the special information about the form of a medication, as provided in the following graphic.

- **Type of med in package**
  - Tablets, capsules, liquids, suppositories, ointments, etc.

- **Abbreviations or words that describe form**
  - CR (controlled release), DS (double-strength)

- **Barcode symbols**
  - Aid in inventory control and distribution
  - Administering the incorrect form of a medication is a medication error!

An additional safety precaution of a medication label involves the bar code. In electronic medical records and the associated use of an electronic MAR, the use of a bar code scanner allows nurses to scan each medication before administering it to the patient. When the medication bar code is scanned, the computer compares the specific medication bar code to the medication order provided in the system, to determine if the nurse is about to administer the correct medication (it is a safety check using a computerized version of the 6 rights!).

Reading the Label: Route

The route should be clearly indicated on the label. Examples include: Oral, IM, IV, topical, optic, otic, and so on. Unless otherwise stated, capsules, pills, and tablets are understood to be oral meds. Liquid medications must be carefully reviewed. The label indicates if a liquid medication needs to be administered orally or by injection. You must follow the exact administration indication. The label also specifically indicates if the medication is a special type as noted earlier. This may include medications with extended action or slow release and as such should NEVER be crushed or chewed. They may be labeled with: CR (controlled release), LA (long acting), EC (enteric coated), or SR (sustained release). A medication that is the same with the exception of the addition of CR, LA, EC, or SR is NOT the same medication and should never be assumed as a substitute.

Reading the Label: Total Volume

Liquid medications list an additional feature not found on other types of medication labels. The medication containers of liquids tell the reader the total volume of the medication supplied in the container. Strength of a liquid medication is expressed as medication per volume of solution (e.g., mg in mL → 5mg per 10mL). Note the total volume and strength in the following image.

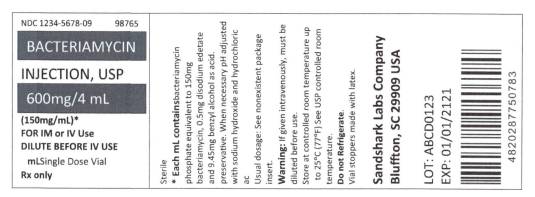

The total volume of the medication in the preceding example is 4mL. The strength of the medication is listed as 150mg/mL. This means that there are 150mg in 1mL of the liquid. If you can quickly do the math in your head, you easily realize that the entire vial of medication contains 600mg of Bacteriamycin in 4mL of solution. This information allows the nurse to compare the medication provided from the pharmacy to the amount of medication ordered and decide not only how much medication to withdraw from the vial but to determine, based on the route, what syringe to use to draw up the medication. In the next chapter we will begin using label information as the basis of refreshing math skills and applying it to everyday clinical situations.

Reading the Label: Amount

The amount of the medication provided in a container involves the solid form of a medication.

The medication amount refers to the total number of capsules or tablets in the total container. In addition, the strength of each tablet or capsule is provided. Do not confuse total volume or total amount in a container with dosage strength.

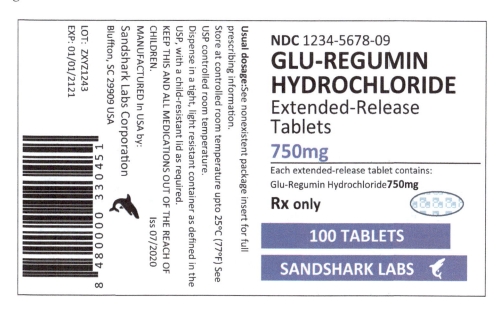

In the preceding label example, note that the medication is a solid form. It is supplied in a tablet. The word tablets is clearly written on the label. In addition, we see that the dosage strength of each tablet is 750mg. The amount of medication contained in the bottle is 100 tablets. As an aside, do you see how the medication also clearly states "extended-release"? This is an indication that the medication should not be crushed or chewed given the special type of tablet contained in the bottle.

Reading the Label: Precautions and Expiration

As noted earlier, if a medication has a special indication or precaution it is provided on the label. In addition, every medication label has an expiration date or a date at which point the manufacturer can no longer guarantee its effectiveness or potency. All medication labels must contain any specific safety information for a medication as well as guidelines for safe handling and storage. The storage directions are equally important because they provide information on how a medication should be stored to prevent the medication from losing its potency or effectiveness. Here are a few common examples: Protect from light; Keep tightly closed; Refrigerate after opening.

Reading the Label: Over the Counter Medications

> SAFETY ALERT!
> ALWAYS CHECK EXPIRATION DATESa

An over the counter medication (OTC) refers to a medication that a person may purchase without a prescription. All safety information, handling, storage, and the recommended frequency and dose are found on the packaging itself. This includes specific medication facts (the name of the medication and its purpose), uses of the medication, warnings and directions of how to take the medication. See the following example. The label represents a common OTC brand name medication with the generic name of the medication provided under it just as we noted in the prescription label.

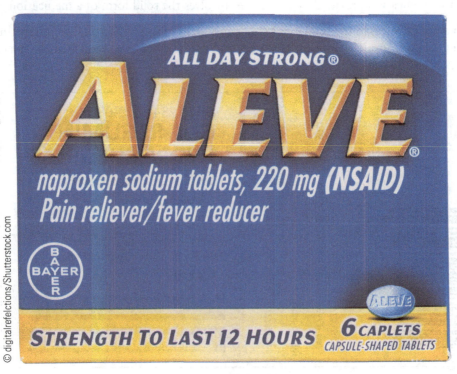

What is the difference between prescription and the OTC medications?

As provided by Byrne (2020),

> Prescription drugs are intended for use by one individual patient to treat a specific condition. Prescription drugs must pass through many clinical trial phases, approval by the FDA and monitored for safety and side effects even after the drug is on the market.
>
> OTC medications are not intended for a specific individual, although depending on the medication, such as creams, eye drops or nasal sprays, the user may want to be the only consumer of the medication. Additionally, OTC drugs are monitored by the FDA, but it is not as strict as the process prescription drugs must go through. Manufacturers are required to make drugs only based on a specific formula with regards to the strength of the drug and they must have FDA approved labeling and FDA specific dosage to be on the market (paras. 1–4).

Forms of Syringes

As we shift now to the forms of available syringes, we must first consider that each syringe type or form has a specific purpose. Learning about each syringe and its intended use ensures safe patient care and demonstrates clinical competency. In the following drawing, notice that there are four types of syringes provided. The description of each syringe is labeled below the diagram. Each syringe once again indicates the total volume it may contain and is marked by a series of calibrated lines along the side. You will learn the appropriate use of each syringe in the nursing program.

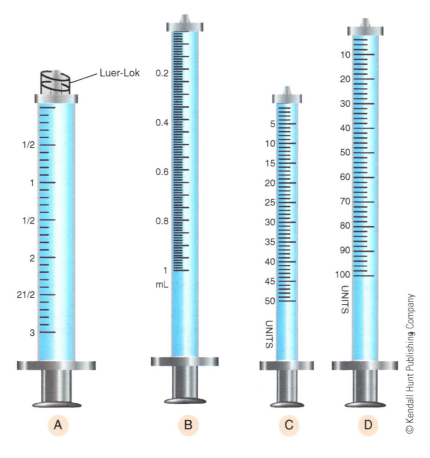

Types of Syringes

(A) Luer-Lok syringe marked in 0.1 (tenths). (B) Tuberculin syringe marked in 0.01 (hundredths) for dosages of less than 1mL. (C) Insulin syringe marked in units (100). (D) Insulin syringe marked in units (50).

For now, let us focus on how to read a syringe so that we can begin working on required math skills for successful nursing practice.

156 Chapter 11 Introduction to Medication Administration

Reading a Syringe

The preceding image provides the anatomy or parts of the syringe. Oral syringes NEVER contain a needle component. If a cannula, or needle, is present on a prepackaged syringe, the syringe will be used for an intramuscular injection or in the process of drawing up medication for the administration of a medication via an intravenous method. Most intravenous systems allow medication to be instilled into the IV tubing through a needleless port. The needle in this case would be removed and the lured hub tip of the syringe would connect to the port of the IV through a locking twist action. There are several sizes of syringes and they are available in 1, 3, 5, 10, 20, 30, and 40mL sizes. The syringes are all calibrated to ensure that the most accurate measurement of medication or solution as ordered has been properly drawn up to be administered. Nurses do not "eye-ball" the amount. We select the correct syringe for the procedure and the amount required and the measurement of the amount, once in the syringe, is exact.

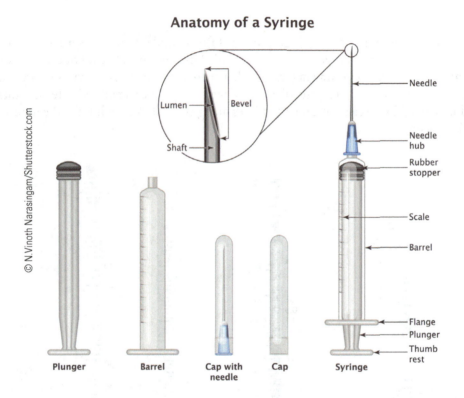

Anatomy of a Syringe

Drawing Up and Interpreting Medication in a Syringe

When drawing up an oral liquid, always place the medication container on a flat surface so that all the air in the container rises to the top. Then insert the oral syringe as demonstrated in the image, slowly pulling back on the plunger until the correct amount of medication is obtained.

When drawing liquid into a syringe for injection the opposite technique is required. Note the picture above. Despite the method one will learn to draw a medication up for administration; it is critical at this point in your training to understand how to interpret the volume in a syringe. Remember that each type of syringe contains a different volume limit and as such, each syringe will be calibrated in different volume increments. The following graphics are provided for you to review. Carefully look at each image noting the difference in calibration and total volume. Use the practice example to ensure comprehension.

Look at the image closely. First, notice that these syringes are calibrated in units. When a syringe is calibrated in units it can only be used for medications that have a dose strength provided in units. Insulin is one such medication. Compare these syringes to the image of the "types of syringes" found previously. Notice that these syringes match type C in the diagram and is specific to insulin. Nurses must, at all times, demonstrate attention

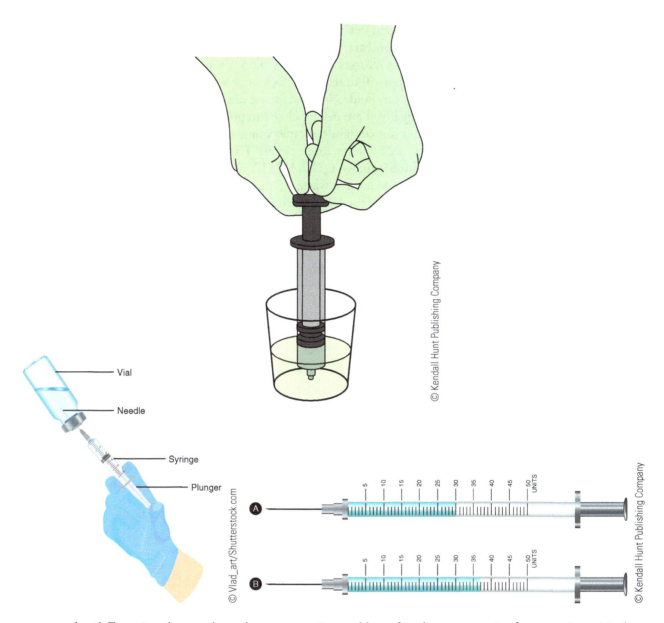

to extreme detail. Ensuring that you have the correct syringe calibrated in the correct unit of measure is a critical detail in preventing medication errors. The preceding image indicates that in syringe A there are 30 units of a liquid medication and in syringe B there are 37 units of a liquid medication. Using the six rights nurses would also ensure that a second RN verifies not only the medication, but the exact amount drawn up in the syringe (without telling the second nurse the total volume) to verify its contents.

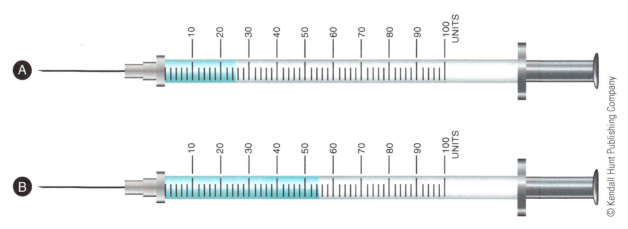

158 Chapter 11 Introduction to Medication Administration

In our second set of images, let us once again determine how many units of medication have been drawn up in each syringe. First, take a moment to compare the two sets of images. In the first set of insulin syringes, what was the total volume that each of the syringes could hold? Did you notice that each one of the syringes in the previous image could only hold up to 50 units? Now look at these set of insulin syringes. What is the total volume that each of these syringes can hold? Note that these are different syringes and can hold up to 100 units. Reading a syringe can be easy if you are paying close attention to the entire situation. While some syringes may be the same size, they may not contain the same volume. Always double check every syringe is critical. In this image, syringe A contains 22.5 units. Look closely. The medication is between the 22 and the 23. It is important to ensure all medication is drawn up EXACTLY as it is ordered. If the order on syringe A's example was for only 22 units, the RN would have to waste 0.5 units of medication to ensure the total volume was exactly 22 units. In syringe example B, the total volume of medication drawn into the syringe is 52 units.

Practice Example 3

Take a moment now to practice reading syringes accurately. The answers are provided for you below the diagram. The unit of measure calibrated on each syringe in the diagram is 1mL.

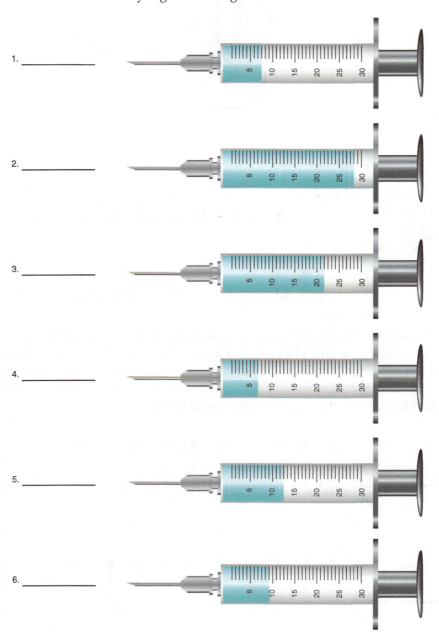

Answers: 1) 11mL, 2) 28mL, 3) 22mL, 4) 7mL, 5) 13mL, 6) 9mL

Summary

The basic skills found in this chapter will help you understand the many steps and safety precautions involved in nursing practice. Your understanding of how to properly interpret an order, especially involving medication administration is critical to being successful in subsequent math calculation competence. Remember, nursing is an art and a science. Until you learn how to artfully care for a patient, you will notice that nursing school is full of rules and safety practices that are exacting and necessary to ensure proper technique and safe patient care. Understanding the various forms of devices used in administering medications, the factors that influence medication dosages, how to properly read a medication label, as well as the common routes and forms of medication are an essential building block to your success.

References

Byrne, M. (2020). *What is the difference between over-the-counter and prescription?* Retrieved from https://www.iwpharmacy.com/blog/difference-between-otc-and-prescription

Food and Drug Administration [FDA]. (2018). *Generic drug facts*. Retrieved from https://www.fda.gov/drugs/generic-drugs/generic-drug-facts

Merriam-Webster. (2020). Meniscus. *Merriam-Webster.com dictionary*. Retrieved from https://www.merriam-webster.com/dictionary/meniscus

Potter, P. A., Perry, A. G., Stockert, P., & Hall, A. (2016). A: *Fundamentals of nursing* (9th ed.). St Louis, MO: Mosby

Chapter 12

Basic Math Review

> **Chapter Objectives:**
> - Understand basic arithmetic functions used in nursing.
> - Demonstrate the proper conversion of roman numerals to whole numbers.
> - Understand fractions and their use in medication orders.
> - Understand decimals and their use in medication orders.
> - Memorize roman numeral and decimal system tables.
> - Discuss the four basic calculation formulas used in medication math calculations.
> - Use practice calculations at the end of the chapter to develop competence and confidence in math used in nursing care.

The review of basic math skills cannot properly begin with thinking about why it is so important that we not only have appropriate math skills, but that we remember them! Let us begin this chapter with a relevant nursing math humor:

> Mike has 72 chocolate bars in his backpack.
> If Mike eats 57 chocolate bars while in nursing class, what does Mike have now?
> Diabetes!! Mike has diabetes!! And probably a stomachache.

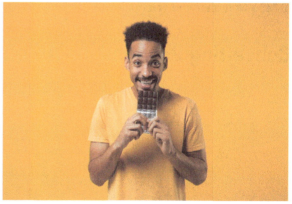

In nursing, calculating the answer to any medication problem involves critical thinking and extreme accuracy. Unlike regular math courses where students may have the impression that everything that they are learning is theoretical and perhaps without real-life application, this is NOT the case with any math required in nursing. Nurses use what is called, "functional math." This is where you take that deep breath! Remember, nurses use math to solve problems for people. It is used to save lives, improve health, and eliminate and prevent infection. We use it to understand medical orders, provide care, and most importantly, ensure we are administering safe, exact doses of all prescribed medication.

This chapter will not review the entirety of what you have learned in formal education but rather review mathematical concepts essential to nursing practice. We begin with the two common numbering systems, Arabic and Roman, used in medication administration.

The Arabic System

The Arabic system uses the numbers 0, 1, 2, 3, 4, 5, 6, 7, 8, and 9. These numbers can be used alone or in combination, as whole numbers, fractions, or decimal numbers (fractions and decimals are described later in this chapter). The Arabic number system is the most common number system used today in nursing, as well as in everyday life.

The Roman System

The Roman system uses selected capital letters such as I, V, X, L, C. These selected capital letters can be changed to "1," "5," "10," "50," "100," in the Arabic system.

Roman Numerals							
1	I	11	XI	30	XXX	500	D
2	II	12	XII	40	XL	600	DC
3	III	13	XIII	50	L	700	DCC
4	IV	14	XIV	60	LX	800	DCCC
5	V	15	XV	70	LXX	900	CM
6	VI	16	XVI	80	LXXX	1,000	M
7	VII	17	XVII	90	XC	2,000	MM
8	VIII	18	XVIII	100	C	3,000	MMM
9	IX	19	XIX	200	CC	4,000	MV
10	X	20	XX	300	CCC	5,000	$\overline{V}$
				400	CD	10,000	$\overline{X}$

These Roman numerals can be combined in accordance with certain rules to represent whole Arabic numbers of "1" and higher and fractions of "1."

Converting Between the Arabic and Roman Systems

> To convert numbers in the Roman system other than single numerals such as "i/I" and "v/V" to numbers in the Arabic system requires adding or subtracting the value of numerals from each other. Whether you add or subtract depends on the values of the numerals and their relative positions.

> *Add* the Arabic values of the numerals when the first Roman numeral is greater than the following numerals.
>
> Example: XII or xii
>
> The X or x represents the Arabic number 10 and the II or ii represents 2.
>
> To convert this number in the Roman system to the Arabic system, add the X (=10) and the II (=2) to get the Arabic equivalent (=12).

> Subtract the Arabic values of the numerals when the first Roman numeral is less than the following numerals.
>
> Example: IX or ix
>
> The I or i represents the Arabic number 1 and the X or x represents the Arabic number 10.
>
> To convert this number in the Roman system to its equivalent in the Arabic system, subtract the I (=1) from the X (=10) to get the Arabic equivalent (=9).

Numbers in the Roman system can be converted to numbers in the Arabic system, as shown in the following table. These conversions must be memorized as nurses must be able to trust their foundational math skills in order to be confident and successful in safe practice.

Roman Number	Arabic Number
I	1
V	5
X	10
L	50
C	100

Why Do Nurses Need to Know Roman Numerals?

In health care, there remain a few medications whose unit of measure involves the apothecary system. While this system was in use for centuries, most medications have been converted to the metric system or household system for administration. According to *Merriam-Webster* (2020), the apothecary system or measure is: "a system of liquid units of measure used chiefly by pharmacists in compounding medical prescriptions that include the gallon, pint, fluid ounce, fluid dram, minim and units of weight such as the grain" (para, 1). Perhaps you have heard of the dram, the ounce, or the scruple? Medication orders are rarely written in the apothecary system but, as always, when an order is written using apothecary units of measure, the RN is professionally responsible for knowing how to calculate the conversion for administration. The few orders that are written in the apothecary system generally use Roman numerals or grains. When used in the apothecary system, Roman numerals may be topped with a horizontal line to prevent the Roman numerals from being mistaken for letters. Also, the Roman numeral "i" or "I" (which is equal to the Arabic "1") is often written in the apothecary system with a dot above the line, as in the following example: gr, $\overline{xi}$, $\overline{vii}$, $\overline{iv}$

Practice Example 1

Let us take a moment for you to practice your ability to properly match the Arabic number with the Roman numeral.

Item	Your Answer	Choices
500		C
10		I
50		V
5		X
100		D
1		L
1,000		M

Ans: 500-D, 10-X, 50-L, 5-V, 100-C, 1-I, 1,000-M

Fractions

A fraction is a way of expressing a part or parts of a whole. A fraction is composed of a numerator and a denominator. All fractions have numerators and denominators. The numerator is always on the top, and the denominator is always on the bottom of the fraction. The denominator represents the total number of parts in the whole. The numerator represents the number of parts of the whole that are present. In the example just given, the whole is divided into six parts (the denominator) and one part (the numerator) is present. The fraction could be read as "one sixth" or as "one of six parts of the whole." Note: A larger denominator means there are more parts in the whole and therefore each individual part is smaller. See how simple that is? ...and you thought fractions were difficult!

$$\text{Example : Fraction} = \frac{1}{6} = \frac{\text{Numerator}}{\text{Denominator}}$$

Practice Example 2

Match the following using the numbers provided next to the numeric fraction in the empty box. The pictures on the left represent the fraction displayed in a visual pie expression or "pieces of a pie." The written numeric fractions are displayed on the right as 2/3rd, 3/4ths, 8/9ths and so on.

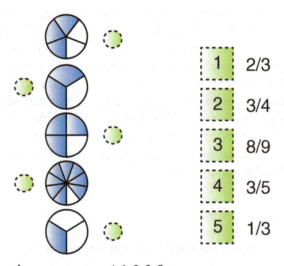

1	2/3
2	3/4
3	8/9
4	3/5
5	1/3

Answer sequence: 4, 1, 2, 3, 5

Identifying Types of Fractions

In nursing we must be able to work through any potential calculation in which any of the 5 common forms of fractions may be used. Let us take a moment to review these common types and an example of each to refresh our memories.

Type of Fraction	Definition	Value	Examples
Proper	Numerator is smaller than denominator	Always less than 1	2/3, 7/8, 15/16
Improper	Numerator is larger than or equal to denominator	Always greater than or equal to 1	3/2, 8/7, 16/15, 3/3
Mixed Number	Whole number followed by a fraction	Always greater than 1	$2\frac{1}{2}$ $4\frac{2}{3}$ $6\frac{7}{8}$
Complex	Numerator, denominator or both are fractions	May be less than, greater than, or equal to 1	$\frac{2/3}{5/6}$, $\frac{4/5}{2\frac{1}{2}}$
Whole Number	Whole numbers can be expressed as fractions with a denominator of 1	Always greater than or equal to 1	$\frac{3}{1}$, $\frac{4}{1}$, $\frac{6}{1}$

Practice Example 3

The type of fraction example is provided on the left. Use the blank box to indicate the correct type of fraction provided using the corresponding number.

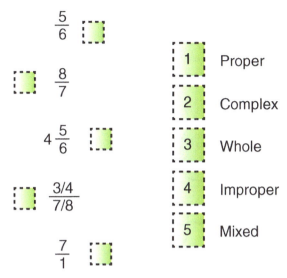

Answer Sequence: 1, 4, 5, 2, 3

Converting a Fraction to a Decimal

The simplest method is to use a calculator. Yes, in nursing school and in practice nurses are allowed to use calculators. In fact, as part of electronic testing, there will be an electronic calculator feature almost always available to you. Just divide the top of the fraction by the bottom and read off the answer! Get your calculator and type in: 5 divided by 8 equals. The answer should be **0.625**. No calculator? It is important with any skill in nursing to know how to calculate or demonstrate the original, or manual version of everything. Even in math. You must be able to competently and easily use long division whenever needed.

Example: here is what long division of 5 divided by 8 looks like:

$$
\begin{array}{r}
0.625 \\
8{\overline{\smash{\big)}\,5.000}} \\
\underline{0} \\
5.0 \\
\underline{4.8} \\
20 \\
\underline{16} \\
40 \\
\underline{40} \\
0
\end{array}
$$

In this example, in order to find the exact answer, it was necessary to insert extra zeros.

Decimals

Many medications are ordered with the use of decimal numbers. The word decimal means "numbered or proceeding by tens." Therefore, decimal numbers are numbers that are multiplied or divided by ten or multiples of ten, such as hundreds and thousands. The numbers to the left of the decimal point are whole numbers, and the numbers to the right of the decimal point are decimal fractions. The decimal point is the "center" of a decimal number. After decimal problems are solved, decimal fractions are rounded off to tenths. If the hundredth column is 5 or greater, the tenth is increased by 1. For example: 0.25 is rounded up to 0.3; 0.24 is rounded to 0.2.

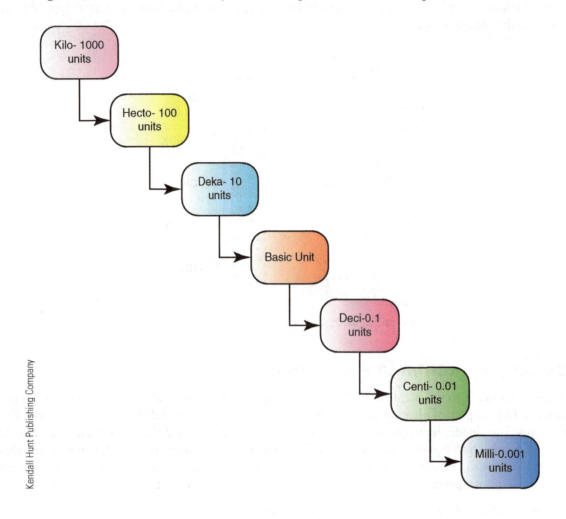

Dosages Written as Decimals

Examples: Here are three medications with dosages written in decimal numbers. At this point in your studies, it is not necessary to know what the medications are. The focus of this chapter is simply to ensure you are competent in basic math skills. You will have an entire course specific to medications called *Pharmacology*, where you will learn about all medications and their properties.

Lanoxin .2mg
Capoten 6.2mg
Synthroid 0.2mg

Let us examine more closely the first example medication and its prescribed dose strength to see how it was written. The goal is to ensure you understand decimals to reduce the possibility of misreading the intended dosage. The medication example Lanoxin .2mg is written incorrectly. Notice that .2mg might be mistaken as 2mg, which would not reflect the intended order. The rule for writing decimals requires that a leading zero is placed before any decimal to accurately indicate that the medication requested is a fraction of a whole. In this way the correct way to write the medication would be 0.2mg.

Decimals Written as Fractions

As we learned in the type of fraction section, decimal numbers can be expressed as fractions in which the denominator is 10 or a multiple of 10 (such as 100 or 1000). Here are some examples of decimal numbers expressed as fractions:

0.45 is 45 hundredths (45/100)
1.25 is 1 and 25 hundredths (1 25/100)
0.6 is 6 tenths (6/10)
0.60 is 60 hundredths or 6 tenths (60/100 or 6/10)
0.054 is 54 thousandths (54/1000)

Notice that the holding place of the last number, after the decimal point, indicates the *number of parts* into which the whole has been divided (tenths, hundredths, or thousandths). To calculate medication dosages accurately, the nurse needs to recognize the place value of numbers written as decimals so that medication can be properly administered. As you may well imagine, when dealing with very small units of measure, providing a patient with 2mL of a medicine would be quite different than providing them with 0.2mL. Something as simple as a misunderstanding of a decimal point place can cause a significant medication error and subsequently cause harm to the patient.

Practice Example 4

Determine the correct place associated with the value of the following decimals. For instance, the decimal 0.01 represents the hundredths place and as a fraction would be written 1/100 of a unit.

0.02	
0.5	
0.11	
0.3	
0.005	
0.011	

Answer: 0.02 = the hundredths place (2/100), 0.5= the tenths place (5/10), 0.11 = the hundredths place (11/100), 0.3= the tenths place (3/10), 0.005 = the thousandths place 5/1000), 0.011 = the thousandths place (11/1000).

Basic Calculation Formulas

In this section, we will review the four methods for calculating drug dosages:

Basic formula
Ratio and proportion
Fractional equation
Dimensional analysis

For the student, it is important to select the formula or method that works for the individual. Once you review the following ways to calculate medications, pick ONE method and stick with it. Do not try to move between the different methods or it will lead to confusion. The goal is to develop competency and thus confidence in your ability to correctly compute math calculations. Take a moment to walk through each method before making your selection.

Method 1: The Basic Formula (BF)

D = dose ordered by physician
H = dose on label of container
V = form and amount in which the drug comes (tablet, capsule, etc.)

This formula is represented as:

$$\frac{D}{H} \times V = \text{Amount to give}$$

Basic Formula Example Problem

Problem 1

Order: Erythromycin 0.5g, PO, q8h
Drug available: 250mg tablets

Hint: Convert grams to milligrams: 0.5g = 500mg

Solve using basic formula

$$\frac{D}{H} \times V = \text{Amount to give}$$

$$\frac{D}{H} \times V = \frac{500}{250} \times 1 \text{ tablet} = 2 \text{ tablets}$$

Answer: Erythromycin 0.5g = 2 tablets

Problem 2

Order: loracarbef (Lorabid) 0.5g, PO, q12h
Drug available: Lorabid 200mg/5mL

Hint: Convert grams to milligrams: 0.5g = 500mg
Solve using basic formula

$$\frac{D}{H} \times V = \text{Amount to give}$$

$$\frac{D}{H} \times V = \frac{500}{200} \times 5\text{mL} = 12.5\text{mL}$$

Answer: Lorabid 0.5g per dose = 12.5mL

Problem 3

Order: Phenobarbital 120mg, STAT
Drug available: Phenobarbital 30mg per tablet

Solve using basic formula

$$\frac{D}{H} \times V = \text{Amount to give}$$

$$\frac{D}{H} \times V = \frac{120}{30} \times 1 = 4 \text{ tablets}$$

Answer: Phenobarbital 120mg = 4 tablets

Problem 4

Order: Meperidine (Demerol) 35mg, IM, STAT
Drug available: Demerol 50mg/mL

Solve using basic formula

$$\frac{D}{H} \times V = \text{Amount to give}$$

$$\frac{D}{H} \times V = \frac{35}{50} \times 1\text{mL} = 0.7\text{mL}$$

Answer: Meperidine (Demerol) 35mg = 0.7mL

Method 2: Ratio and Proportion (RP)

Now let us look at another method for calculating. Ratio and proportion simply involves what is known and what is desired using a method setting up the problem that resembles a table and ratio indicators. The [:] or the [::] respectively.

```
       Known                    Desired
   H   :   V        ::       D     :     X
on hand : vehicle   ::  desired dose : amount to give
```

H and V: known quantities—dose on hand and vehicle

D and X: desired dose and unknown amount to give

Multiply the means and the extremes

Solve for X

Problem 1

Order: Erythromycin 0.5g, PO, q8h
Drug available: 250mg tablets

Hint: Convert grams to milligrams: 0.5g = 500mg

Solve using ratio and proportion

```
       Known                    Desired
   H  :  V       ::       D    :    X
on hand : vehicle ::  desired dose : amount to give
```

H	:	V	::	D	:	X
250mg	:	1 tab		500mg	:	X tab
		250 X	=	500		
		X	=	2 tablets		

Answer: Erythromycin 0.5g = 2 tablets

Problem 2

Order: Aspirin (ASA) 650mg × PRN
Drug available: Aspirin 325mg/tablet

Solve using ratio and proportion

```
       Known                    Desired
   H  :  V       ::       D    :    X
on hand : vehicle ::  desired dose : amount to give
```

H	:	V	::	D	:	X
325mg	:	1 tab		650mg	:	X tab
		325 X	=	650		
		X	=	2 tablets		

Answer: Aspirin 650mg = 2 tablets

Problem 3

Order: amoxicillin 75mg, PO, qid
Drug available: 125mg/5mL oral suspension

Solve using ratio and proportion

```
       Known                    Desired
   H  :  V       ::       D    :    X
on hand : vehicle ::  desired dose : amount to give
```

H	:	V	::	D	:	X
125mg	:	5mL		75mg	:	XmL
		125 X	=	375		
		X	=	3ML		

Answer: Amoxicillin 75mg = 3mL

Method 3: Fractional Equation (FE)

The third method used by nurses to solve medication calculations involves fractional equation or what is more commonly known as algebra. Take a look at the following:

$$\frac{H}{V} = \frac{D}{X}$$

H = dosage on hand or in the container
V = vehicle or form in which the drug comes
D = desired dosage
X = unknown amount to give

The fractional equation is the most common form of nursing calculation because the prerequisite math coursework for every nursing program is the successful completion of Algebra I and II. Students readily understand the use of Algebra and most students choose to always set up their medication calculations using this method.

Problem 1

Order: Erythromycin (ERY-TAB) 750mg, PO, q8h
Drug available: Erythromycin (ERY-TAB) 250mg tablets

Solve using fractional equation

$$\frac{H}{V} = \frac{D}{X}$$

$$\frac{H}{V} = \frac{D}{X} \quad \frac{250\text{mg}}{1 \text{ tablet}} = \frac{750\text{mg}}{X}$$

$$250 = 750$$
$$x = 3$$

Answer: Erythromycin 750mg = 3 tablets

Problem 2

Order: valproic acid (Depakene) 100mg, PO, tid
Drug available: 250mg/5mL oral suspension

Solve using fractional equation

$$\frac{H}{V} = \frac{D}{X}$$

$$\frac{H}{V} = \frac{D}{X} \quad \frac{250\text{mg}}{5\text{mL}} = \frac{100}{X}$$

$$250\,X = 500$$
$$X = 2\text{mL}$$

Answer: Valproic acid 100mg = 2mL

Problem 3

Order: atropine 0.6mg, IM, STAT
Drug available: 0.4mg per mL

Solve using fractional equation

$$\frac{H}{V} = \frac{D}{X}$$

$$\frac{H}{V} = \frac{D}{X} \quad \frac{0.4\text{mg}}{1\text{mL}} = \frac{0.6\text{mg}}{X}$$

$$X = 0.6$$

$$X = 1.5\text{mL}$$

Answer: atropine 0.6mg = 1.5mL

Method 4: Dimensional Analysis (DA)

The use of dimensional analysis reflects a recent education method in K-12 in solving multiple step problems. Again, you, as the learner, must decide which method you will use in solving medication calculation equations and stick with that method. Dimensional analysis separates a problem into three factors, the drug label factor, the conversion factor, and the drug order factor. Let us take a look at dimensional analysis:

Calculates dosages with three factors

Drug label factor: form of drug dose (V) with its equivalence in units (H)

(e.g., 1 capsule = 500mg)

Conversion factor (C): memorize conversions such as 1g = 1,000mg and 1mg = 1,000mcg

Drug order factor: dosage desired (D)

$$V \text{ (form of drug)} = \frac{V \text{ (form of drug)} \times D \text{ (desired dose)}}{H \text{ (on hand)} \times 1 \text{ or blank}}$$

(drug label)   (drug order)

$$V \text{ (form of drug)} = \frac{V \text{ (drug form)} \times C \text{ (H)} \times D \text{ (desired dose)}}{H \text{ (on hand)} \times C \text{ (D)} \times 1 \text{ or blank}}$$

(drug label)   (conversion factor) (drug order)

Now let us try a similar drug calculation problem as in our previous method examples to see the dimensional analysis method at work.

Problem 1

Order: Erythromycin (ERY-TAB) 1g, PO, q12h
Drug available: Erythromycin (ERY-TAB) 250mg tablets

**Drug ordered and dosage on bottle are in metric system, but notice that the units differ

Conversion Factor: 1.0g = 1000mg

Solve using dimensional analysis

$$\text{tab} = \frac{1\text{ tab} \times 1000\text{mg} \times 1\text{g}}{250\text{mg} \times 1\text{g} \times 1}$$

$$1\text{ tab} \times 4 = 4\text{ tabs}$$

Answer: Erythromycin 1g = 4 tablets

Problem 2

Order: acetaminophen (Tylenol) 1gram, PO, PRN
Drug available: 325mg tablets

Conversion Factor: 1000mg = 1g
Solve using dimensional analysis

$$\text{Tab} = \frac{1\text{ tab} \times 100\text{mg} \times 1\text{gram}}{325\text{mg} \times 1\text{gram} \times 1} = \frac{1000}{325} = 3.07\text{ tab or 3 tablets}$$

Answer: Acetaminophen 1g = 3 tablets

Problem 3

Order: ciprofloxacin (Cipro) 500mg, PO, q12h
Drug available: 250mg tablets

Solve using dimensional analysis

$$\frac{1\text{ tab} \times 500\text{mg}}{250\text{mg} \times 1} = 2\text{ tablets}$$

Answer: Ciprofloxacin 500mg = 2 tablets

Summary

In this chapter, you reviewed the basic arithmetic functions used in solving medication calculations. By reviewing both Arabic and Roman numerals, you discovered that many medications are based in Roman numeral units based on the apothecary system. These basic rules led to the discovery and explanation of the four common methods for drug calculations: the basic formula, ratio and proportion, fractional equation and dimensional analysis. Each student learner is responsible for determining which calculation method most easily conforms to his learning style and adopt it as his sole method for calculation.

References

Merriam-Webster.com. (2020). Apothecaries' measure [definition]. Retrieved from https://www.merriam-webster.com/dictionary/apothecaries%27%20measure

Chapter 13

Frequently Used Systems of Measurement

Chapter Objectives:

- Express metric measures correctly using rules of the metric system.
- State common equivalents in the metric system and convert measures within the metric system.
- Differentiate apothecary and household system of measurement.
- Identify reasons for nonuse of apothecary measures and symbols.
- State the common household equivalents & specific household system rules.
- Identify measures in the household system.
- Define other measures used in medication administration and state the equivalent metric and household approximate equivalents.
- Convert a unit of measure to its equivalent within the same system
- Convert a unit from one system of measurement to its equivalent in another system of measurement.
- Convert between Celsius and Fahrenheit temperature.
- Convert between units of length: inches, centimeters, and millimeters.
- Convert between units of weight: pounds and kilograms, pounds and ounces to kilograms.
- Convert between traditional and international time.

In this chapter, multiple systems of measurement will be explored and applied to nursing practice. The concepts found in the chapter will, once again, require constant repetitive use and memorization to ensure competency in nursing school and beyond. As a nurse, you will be required to easily convert between systems of measurement in everyday clinical practice. This includes converting time, weight, and basic conversion between systems such as is involved in calculating a patient's intake and output and dosing medication.

Systems of Measurement

Metric System

- Preferred system of measurement in the health care setting
- Also known as International System of Units or SI units (from Systéme International d'Unités)
- Simple and accurate because it is based on the decimal system
- The metric system should be used to prevent medication errors
- Decimal system—multiples of ten (10)

Chapter 13 Frequently Used Systems of Measurement

- Three basic units of measure:
    - Gram (weight)—measure medications as solids
    - Liter (volume)—measure medications as solutions
    - Meter (length)—measure body parts, wounds, etc.
- Prefixes—memorization is necessary
    - Kilo, centi, milli, micro
- Name of basic unit is incorporated into measure
    - Milli*liter*, kilo*gram*, centi*meter*

Basic Units of Metric Measurement		
Table of Measure	Basic Unit	Abbreviation
Weight (solid)	Gram	g
Volume (liquid)	Liter	L
Length	Meter	m

Examples of use of prefixes and suffixes
67 milligrams
milli = thousandths, grams = unit of weight—therefore,
67 milligrams = 67 thousandths of a gram
Milliliter = one thousandth portion of a liter
Kilogram = one thousand grams
Deciliter = one tenth of a liter
Cubic millimeter = mm3 (length × width × height)
Used to count blood cells in fixed volume on slides
Abbreviations are first letter of the word

Gram = g
Meter = m
Liter = L (capital letter)

When prefixes are used with basic units, the first letter of the word is written in lower case

Milligram = mg
Microgram = mcg
Exception—Liter as in milliliter = mL

A mnemonic to help remember the important metric prefixes order from largest measurement to smallest. Here is an example but you are welcome to create your own!

Kitty	Hawk	Doesn't	Drink	Canned	Milk	Much
kilo	hecto	deka	deci	centi	milli	micro

Common Metric Abbreviations
gram—g
microgram—mcg
milligram—mg
kilogram—kg
liter—L
deciliter—dL (seen in the report of lab values)
milliliter—mL

As noted in our previous chapters there are very specific safety rules when using decimals and they include the following:

Safe Practice Table
Arabic number expresses quantity (1, 0.5)
Parts or fractions of a whole are expressed as decimals (0.4 g NOT 2/5g)
Quantity precedes unit of measure (2L)
A full space is used between number and abbreviation (5mg)
Use leading zero before a decimal, but eliminate trailing zeros (0.4mg NOT .4mg, and 2mg NOT 2.0mg)
DO NOT USE mu symbol "μ" with grams, write mcg NOT "µg"
DO NOT USE "cc" for mL
2mL NOT 2 cc
(Why do we no longer use "cc"?)
It can easily be misinterpreted as 00. Be cognizant of this as some syringes may still be calibrated in "cc"
The "cc" may still be seen on some syringes
Place commas in values starting at one thousand (ISMP recommendation) 1,000 NOT 1000
Do not add "s" to make plurals—could lead to misinterpretation mg NOT mgs
Safety Point: These rules are designed to prevent medication errors and ensure accurate interpretation of metric annotations used in medication administration.

Metric Units of Measured Weight Reminders

Gram—basic unit of weight

Milligrams and micrograms are multiple times smaller than a gram

1g = 1,000mg therefore, 1g = 1,000,000mcg

Kilogram is the only unit typically used in medicine that is larger than the basic gram unit (used to measure client weight)

1,000g = 1kg—so 1kg is 1,000 times larger than 1g

Metric Units of Measured Volume Reminders

In volume, the Liter is the basic unit of volume. The milliliter (mL) is much smaller than a liter.

1L = 1,000mL, and 1mL is 0.001 of a liter

Reminder: "cc" or cubic centimeter is no longer accepted by The Joint Commission (TJC).

Pints and quarts (used in home care) are not metric but have metric equivalents.

1 quart ≈ 1,000mL and 1 pint ≈ 500mL

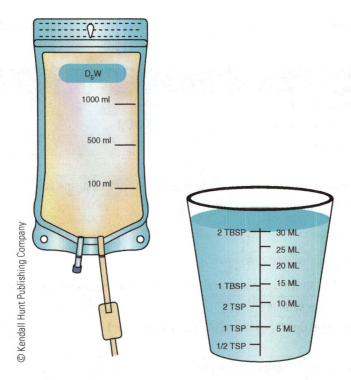

Note that in nursing, many of the medications provided to patients are in a liquid form requiring nurses to have an acute sense of a liquid measure. Where nurses are measuring: 1) how much someone has consumed, 2) measuring a patient output, or 3) pouring an oral liquid medication or administering IV fluids, it is imperative that fluid volume make sense. In the preceding images, you recognize the medication cup, calibrated on the side with both metric volume and household measures. IV fluids, on the other hand, exclusively come in metric volume measures which form the foundation of what is known as an *IV calculation*. Later in the program you will learn how to calculate the rate of an IV medication and use the drip factor to determine the number of drops per minute.

Conversions Between Systems

Convert means to change from one unit to another, such as mg to mcg. This is accomplished by moving the decimal. Move the decimal *Left* to divide and *Right* to multiply.

Conversion factors: 1kg = 1,000g 1g = 1,000mg 1mg = 1,000mcg 1L = 1,000mL

To convert a smaller number to a larger number—DIVIDE—move the decimal to the *left*. Here is an example:

    100mL = ___ L   (Conversion Factor: 1,000mL = 1L)
    (smaller) (larger)

    Move decimal 3 places to left: 100 = 0.1L

To convert a larger number to a smaller number—MULTIPLY—move the decimal to the *right*. Here is an example: 0.75g = ___ mg (Conversion Factor: 1g = 1,000mg)
    (larger) (smaller)

Move decimal 3 places to right: 0.750 = 750mg

Did you remember to do that correctly? Practice makes perfect so try the following practice example on your own.

Practice Example 1

Convert the following metric measures:

a. 400mg = _____ mcg

b. 49mL = _____ L

c. 3.75L = _____ mL

d. 0.08kg = _____ g

Answer: a. 400,000 mcg, b. 0.049L, c. 3,750mL, d. 80g

Apothecary

The first question that many students ask when it comes to the Apothecary system is: Where did this come from? Chance s are that you did not learn this in school but it has been around for centuries. As discussed in the last chapter, the apothecary system has an English origin and was at one time also referred to as the *fraction system*. Over time, the symbols and use of roman numerals became confusing and slowly measurement systems have changed over to metric measurement. Despite TJC recommending that all apothecary measures be removed and replaced on their "Do Not Use" list, some medications are still formulated using this old system of measurement. Your role as the professional RN will always be to convert these medication amounts to the metric system as accurately as possible to avoid error. Within this system, nurses need to know these basic essential conversions:

Volume

1 pint = 16 fluid ounces
1 quart = 32 fluid ounces = 2 pints

Weight

Grain = gr

> Safety Note: Be careful not to confuse grain (gr) with gram (g)

Grains are written with the measure before the amount, example: grXV which means 15 grains. We know the conversion of grains to grams and milligrams. The trick is to remember the face of a clock. The clock has 60 minutes. Let the 60 minutes be represented as milligrams in this illustration. 60mg is roughly 1 grain (written as grI). Think this through—if 1 grain is 60 milligrams then how many grains would 30mg be? The answer is ½ of a grain or gr1/2. How about a 15mg? 15 milligrams represent ¼ of a grain or gr1/4.

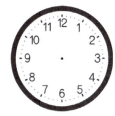

Apothecary System Notes to Know!

Metric equivalents: *gr15 = 1g* and *gr1 = 60–65 mg (technically)*; however, most meds are based on the equivalent gr1 = 60mg

Volume

Ounce = oz
Metric equivalent: 1oz = 30mL
Medicine cups are 1oz capacity

Household Measurement

Household is a measurement system that you should already be familiar with in your home. In fact, it is used every single day in the kitchen, especially when making recipes. Household measurement represents one of the oldest and least accurate systems because it is based on glass containers and utensils which are not scientific in nature. Their capacity varies based on the manufacturer who may be more concerned with how a product looks than accuracy of measurement. To test your household measuring cups and measuring spoons, use a dropper or syringe to determine their volume. It is important therefore to memorize the following conversion for nursing school in addition to the conversions in the table found in the next section. One very important fact regarding the household system of measure is that the smallest unit of measure is that of the drop represented by the following abbreviation (gtt). In nursing you will learn to calculate the drip rate (or the number of drops) of an IV fluid for accurate administration of a particular volume to a patient.

Memorize:

$$1 \text{ teaspoon (t, tsp)} = 5\text{mL}$$
$$1 \text{ tablespoon (T, tbs)} = 15\text{mL}$$
$$1 \text{ measuring cup (c)} = 8\text{oz}$$

Conversions

A conversion simply means, changing from one form to another. This can be accomplished within the same system (e.g., mg to mcg) or between systems (e.g., oz to mL). While we are approximating the result, continuity exists in the conversions. Converting is a necessary skill used to administer the ordered amount of medication. Remember our medicine cup once again.

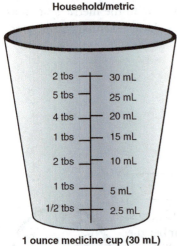

1 ounce medicine cup (30 mL)

Notice that it is calibrated in both household and metric units for easy conversion and use in the clinical setting.

Now it is time to memorize. As you might have guessed, in order to be successful there are several basic conversions that must be committed to memory for quick recall. You will be expected to move between household and metric equivalents on a daily basis in nursing. Additionally, DO NOT use online conversion calculators or tables found on the Internet. Use ONLY the conversion tables provided to you in class. The following table aligns with these measurement requirements. Equivalents are not exact, but the memorization of equivalents is essential for proficiency in medication administration and in ensuring that patients can safely self-administer medications. It is important to learn equivalents before using conversions.

UNIT	Abbreviation	Equivalent	Metric Equivalent
teaspoon	t (tsp)	------------	5mL
tablespoon	T (tbs)	1T = 3T	15mL
ounce (fluid)	oz	1oz = 2T	30mL
cup (standard measuring)	C	1 cup = 8oz	240mL
pint	pt	1pt = 2 cups (16oz)	500mL
quart	qt	1qt = 4 cups = 2pt = 32oz	1,000mL
pound (weight)	lb	1lb = 16oz	2.2lb = 1kg (1,000g)
inch	in	------------	1in = 2.5cm or 0.25m

Practice in your own kitchen using the measuring spoons and measuring cups for household cooking and baking. Take a moment to also watch the following videos found under this textbook's video collection for chapter 13. Metric and Household Measures Demonstrated for Nursing: https://youtu.be/qzeJsGDxi9Q. From www.Registerednursern.com: What is the metric table for nursing calculations? https://youtu.be/aGMLRnWGanM. Putting in the amount of work it will require to memorize and easily mentally convert measurement may be very easy for you or may be a bit more difficult depending on your foundation in math and science. The real answer is to stick with it! The more you practice, the easier conversions will become.

Moving Decimals

There is another way to visually remember how to convert using decimals. Remember: When moving from a smaller to a larger number, move the decimal to the left.

$$350\text{mg} = 0.35\text{g}$$

Remember to always place a zero (0) in front of the decimal point to indicate a value that is less than 1. When moving a decimal from a larger number to a smaller number, move the decimal to the right.

$$0.850\text{L} = 850\text{mL}$$

Other Important Units of Measurement

There are a few other measurements that are used in dosage calculations that are helpful to learn in the beginning. These measures will allow you to easily calculate medication problems because you will recognize the unit associated with the dose.

These include:

Units: amount of medication in 1 mL of solution. Units measure specific medications in terms of action (examples: heparin, penicillin, and insulin).

International Units: unit of potency. *IU* represents the amount that is needed to produce a certain effect (examples: vitamins, chemicals).

Milliequivalents (mEq): used to measure electrolytes and ionic activity of a medication. A milliequivalent represents one thousandth of the equivalent weight of an ion (examples: potassium, calcium).

Practice Example 2

Test your conversion knowledge by answering the following:

1. 16oz = _____ cup
2. 2pts = _____ mL
3. 60mL = _____ oz
4. 45mL = _____ tbs

Which unit of measurement should not be abbreviated?

1. Drops (gtt)
2. Unit (U)
3. Milliequivalent (mEq)
4. Pound (lb)
5. Kilograms (kg)

Ans: 1) 2 cups, 2) 1,000mL, 3) 2oz, 4) 3tb

Temperature Conversions

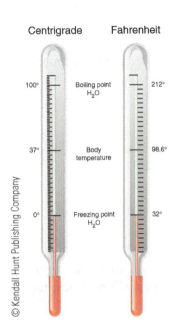

Have you ever wondered why the United States teaches and uses Fahrenheit to measure temperature? Did you know that most other countries report temperature using Celsius? While that is a topic for a history class, it is important to know both systems in nursing. Because nurses need to know both systems, there are two *very easy* conversion methods that will aid you. While a nurse can set a thermometer to read in both a °F or a °C format, recorded temperatures in the medical record are generally required in the Celsius measure.

There are a few basics that must be readily understood with regard to temperature. First, a numeric temperature, followed a °F indicates that the reading is in Fahrenheit. A numeric temperature followed by a °C indicates that the reading is in Celsius. To keep temperatures straight in your head, it may be helpful to memorize two specific facts in case you become confused in which direction to convert a temperature between the two systems. The freezing point of water is 32 degrees F or 0 degrees C. The boiling point of water is 212 degrees F or 100 degrees C. Note the following graphic comparing the two different measures of temperature.

Take a moment now to make these two simple equations stick in your mind. Examples of each conversion have been provided.

To convert from Celsius to Fahrenheit, multiply by 1.8 and add 32

Example: Convert 37.5°C to °F

Formula:

$$°F = 1.8(°C) + 32$$

$$°F = (1.8 \times 37.5) + 32$$

$$°F = 67.5 + 32$$

$$°F = 99.5°$$

To convert from Fahrenheit to Celsius, subtract 32 and divide by 1.8.

Example: Convert 68°F to °C

Formula:

$$°C = (°F - 32) \div 1.8$$

$$°C = (68 - 32) \div 1.8$$

$$°C = 36 \div 1.8$$

$$°C = 20°$$

Conversions: Metrics and Length

Another interesting fact in American culture is our insistence on the use of the Imperial system. This should not be a complete surprise as the Imperial system came from the British and the United States has a significant history with this empire. The Imperial system comprises of the mile, while the Metric system uses the kilometer. The Imperial system uses the pound and the Metric system uses the kilogram. Because of this, the focus of this section is to ensure that the student nurse is equally informed on the use of the metric system for length. In the Imperial system the inch is used but across all health care facilities the proper measurement for length is the Metric centimeter. Let us discuss a few common uses of the metric system for length in clinical practice. Metric measures are used for:

Pupil size expressed in mm
Baby's head circumference expressed in cm
Wounds and incisions
(length × width × depth in cm)

Remember that the conversion factor is extremely important for every medication calculation involving different units of measure. Every student should become comfortable immediately writing down the conversion table or conversion factors on homework and exams until you feel comfortable and confident with your math skill set. Let us walk through an example together using length.

Using the conversion factor: 1cm = 10mm

If incision is 25cm, how many mm is it?

Think to yourself, a mm is smaller, and a cm is larger. In this instance I need to divide by 10 or move the decimal point one place to the left. The resulting equation would look as follows:

$$25mm = 25 \div 10 = 2.5cm \text{ or } 25 = 2.5cm$$

Using the conversion factor: 1in. = 2.5cm
Convert 30cm to inches (in.)

Think to yourself, in this instance I am moving from a smaller unit to a larger unit so I need to divide. The resulting equation would look as follows: 30 ÷ 2.5 = 12in. Did you get this correct?

Weight Conversions

Body weight is important in calculating doses for certain medications delivered in mg or mcg per kilogram. Nurses need to determine and administer medication dosages accurately and safely. To do this, you may need to convert pounds and ounces in pediatric medication calculations. Recall in the previous chapter that all medication calculations involving children will be based on the accurate weight of the child at the time of the prescription. Weight conversions must be accurate to avoid what could be very dangerous errors. In the United States, weight is measured using the pound, but all health care systems record weight using the metric system. This requires nurses to be able to find the metric equivalent or vice versa when weighing any person. For instance, you may be weighing a newborn and you are in luck! The scale in the office is calibrated in grams and kilograms. Just then a parent looks at the resulting weight of her child and says, "That's an odd number, what is her weight in pounds?" This is a great example that happens everyday. You will not be able to escape conversions so you need to go ahead and learn how to confidently remember each factor. To convert pounds to kilograms, remember one simple conversion: 2.2lb is equal to 1kg. If you can remember this, you will note that the way to convert a weight in pounds is to divide the pound result value by 2.2. It is that easy!

Example: Convert 65lb to kilograms

65lb ÷ 2.2 = 29.54kg and that number *rounds to* 29.5kg

When you encounter a situation in which the weight is recorded in pounds *and* ounces, the simple way to convert this to kilograms is to convert the ounces to the nearest tenth of a lb pound and add it to the pounds value. We know that 16oz equals 1lb. Let us try converting a weight in pounds and ounces to kilograms.

Example:

A child weighs: 10lb 2oz, Think: smaller to larger

$$oz \div 16 = 0.12 \text{ which } rounds\ to\ 0.1lb$$

$$10lb + 0.1lb = 10.1lb. \text{ Again, think smaller to larger}$$

$$10.1 \div 2.2 = 4.59 \ rounds\ to\ 4.6\ kg$$

Now that we understand the easy conversion of pounds to kilograms, let us reverse the process and convert kilograms to pounds! I know you would like to say, no thank you at this point, but our learning must continue. This is equally easy to remember. When converting kilograms to pounds we multiply by 2.2 (larger to smaller). Remember one simple conversion: 1kg = 2.2lb so to complete the conversion we will multiply.

Let us try an example:

A child weighs 24.7kg

Convert the 24.7kg to pounds

$$24.7kg \times 2.2 = 54.34lb, \text{ this } rounds\ to\ 54.3lb$$

No matter what you do in nursing you will need to remember weight conversions. After spending years working in the nursery the easiest way to remember whether you multiply, or divide can come down to one simple fact that you choose to remember. We know for instance that a 9-pound baby is exactly 4.082kg or 4,082grams. Done. Remember this static. No matter how confused you may become, if you remember this exact fact in weight you can work your conversion until you decide if you should multiply or divide to obtain the opposite value. Note 4.082 × 2.2 is how much? Roughly 9lb. What if I divided 4.082 by 2.2? The result is 1.855lb. This is not even close! Have you ever held a 9 pound baby? It would immediately make sense that dividing and obtaining a weight of 1.855lb for a good size baby would not be correct. I hope the tip helps!

Military Time

Military time is so named for its use in the military; however, it is officially known as the International time measurement. While most of us are used to measuring time using a 12-hour clock, military time uses a 24-hr clock. In health care, you guessed it! A 24-hour clock is used to help prevent errors by eliminating repetition of numbers. Here are a few important facts to remember regarding military time. (1) despite using a colon when expressing time using a 12-hour clock (ex: 7:00 a.m.) in military time a colon is NEVER used and neither are the a.m. or p.m. designations. (2) When using a 24-hour clock, the concept of midnight or 2400 can easily be confused with the beginning of the next day or 0000; these two times are the same. The difference is simply whether you are saying at midnight 2400 tonight or at 0000 tomorrow morning. Midnight = 0000 and 2400 so be careful to clarify the context. As the clock is a 24-hour clock, note that time in the military system continues past 12 noon on the diagram below. Following 1200 is 1300 which represents 1:00 p.m. and so forth. Here is an example: 7:00 a.m. is written as 0700, whereas 7:00 p.m. is written as 1900.

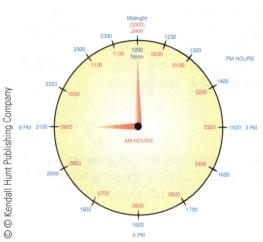

Converting Between Standard Time and International (Military Time)

To convert a.m. time, omit the colon and "a.m.," then add a zero to the beginning to make a four-digit number. For example: 8:45 a.m. = 0845. To convert p.m. time, omit the colon and "p.m.," then add 1200 to the time. For example: 7:50 p.m. = 1950. To convert times between 0000 and 1200, delete any zero at the beginning, insert colon, and add "a.m." For example: 0845 = 8:45 a.m.. To convert times between 1200 and 2400, subtract 1200, insert colon, and add "p.m."

For example: 1950 = 7:50 p.m. Need more help? There are wonderful, quick videos in the chapter video collection that demonstrate these easy conversions! See:

From Registerednursern.com

What is the metric table for nursing calculations? https://youtu.be/aGMLRnWGanM

Grains Nursing Dosage Calculation Problems https://youtu.be/z97PbnvW7CY

Celsius to Fahrenheit Conversion Formula https://youtu.be/wIPsIgVzLkk

Learn Military Time, Quick and Easy: from Airport Travel and Tourism: https://youtu.be/ghOY0x6me_o

You can also access the military practice sheet in chapter resources to text your conversion skills.

Let us now look at a practice example that includes a few of each form of conversion learned in this chapter to test your knowledge. Complete the following example and verify your answers at the end.

Practice Example 3

The following conversions include temperature, weight, and length. Test your memory of these conversions and write the correct answer in the blank portion below.

1. 40°C = ___°F
2. 98.6°F = ___°C
3. 67cm = ___ mm
4. 5 in. = ___ cm
5. 31lb, 7oz = ___ kg

Answer: 104°F, 2) 37°C, 3) 670mm, 4) 12.5cm, 5) 14.29kg

Summary

In summary, you have reviewed basic math skills, medication calculation formulas, and now you have reviewed systems of measurement. Reviewing and, perhaps in some instances, relearning these conversions will serve you well and build your confidence and competence in nursing practice. No matter what field within nursing you may pursue, the creation of solid math skills and the understanding that these skills are simply a function of our roles in delivering safe care should offer you the incentive to master these and future skills in your nursing career. Use every resource available in the textbook to your advantage. You are, after all, the future of nursing and you should begin by demanding nothing but complete excellence and quality from yourself. Remember always that nursing IS an art and a science.

References

Clayton, B. D., & Willihnganz, M. (2017). *Basic pharmacology for nurses* (17th ed.). St. Louis, MO: Mosby.

Kee, J. L., & Marshall, S. M. (2013). *Clinical calculations: With applications to general and specialty areas* (7th ed.). St. Louis, MO: Saunders.